Questions and Answers

FOR THE

Diploma in Occupational Medicine

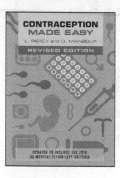
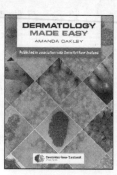
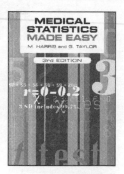
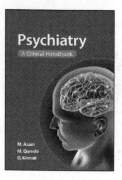
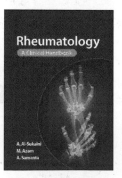
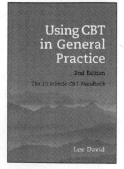

Questions and Answers
FOR THE
Diploma in Occupational Medicine
REVISED EDITION

Clare Fernandes
MBBS, BSc, DRCOG, DOccMed

GP REGISTRAR IN MILTON KEYNES

EDITED BY:
Karen Nightingale
MBChB, BAO, DFPH, DipLSHTM, PGDip, MPH, MFOM

CONSULTANT IN OCCUPATIONAL MEDICINE,
OCCUPATIONAL HEALTH MEDICAL LTD, WARRINGTON

© Scion Publishing Limited, 2017

Revised edition published 2017

First edition (ISBN 978 1 907904 87 5) published in 2016

A CIP catalogue record for this book is available from the British Library.

ISBN 978 1 911510 07 9

Scion Publishing Limited

The Old Hayloft, Vantage Business Park, Bloxham Road, Banbury OX16 9UX, UK
www.scionpublishing.com

Important Note from the Publisher

The information contained within this book was obtained by Scion Publishing Ltd from sources believed by us to be reliable. However, while every effort has been made to ensure its accuracy, no responsibility for loss or injury whatsoever occasioned to any person acting or refraining from action as a result of information contained herein can be accepted by the authors or publishers.

Readers are reminded that medicine is a constantly evolving science and while the authors and publishers have ensured that all dosages, applications and practices are based on current indications, there may be specific practices which differ between communities. You should always follow the guidelines laid down by the manufacturers of specific products and the relevant authorities in the country in which you are practising.

Although every effort has been made to ensure that all owners of copyright material have been acknowledged in this publication, we would be pleased to acknowledge in subsequent reprints or editions any omissions brought to our attention.

Registered names, trademarks, etc. used in this book, even when not marked as such, are not to be considered unprotected by law.

Typeset by Medlar Publishing Solutions Pvt Ltd, India
Printed in the UK by 4edge Limited

Contents

Preface to the revised edition

When I was sitting the DOccMed there were no revision books to aid my study, so I wrote my own. This book is an amalgamation and an extension of the notes I created at the time. They have all been edited by an experienced Consultant in Occupational Health, Dr Karen Nightingale, to whom I owe many thanks.

The book has been written to help you prepare for the written part of the examination and is organized into subject areas rather than as practice exam papers. This is so that you can concentrate your revision on the areas that you need most. Like me, you may find the clinical areas covered are ones that are still familiar from medical school, whereas the specifics of ethics and the law, and the principles relating to occupational health, are entirely new concepts; you will probably have come across only a few of them in your time working in general practice and other specialties and so they will require further attention. I have made a conscious effort to include more questions on the topics that I and my exam cohort found most difficult. The questions are designed to aid your learning and so are generally single best answers.

To try to replicate the exam format, we have also included (as *Chapter 5*) a mock exam written in the style of the exam, where there is more than one potentially correct answer, but only one answer that is the best fit.

Remember that you are not required to know every specific detail to the level of a specialist, and remember that the exam focuses on making sure that those who pass will be safe occupational health providers.

Good luck!

Dr Clare Fernandes MBBS, BSc, DRCOG, DOccMed

April 2017

Acknowledgments

My thanks go to Dr K. Nightingale and Mr B. Pryor.

List of abbreviations

ADL	activities of daily living
ALA	5-aminolevulinic acid
ALARP	as low as is reasonably practicable
ART	assessment of repetitive tasks
BMI	body mass index
CABG	coronary artery bypass graft
CE	Conformité Européenne
COPD	chronic obstructive pulmonary disease
COSHH	Control of Substances Hazardous to Health
CT	computed tomography
DDA	Disability Discrimination Act
DSE	display screen equipment
DVLA	Driver and Vehicle Licensing Agency
EAV	exposure action values
EC	European Commission
ELV	exposure limit values
EPP	exposure-prone procedure
FEV1	forced expiratory volume in 1 second
FOM	Faculty of Occupational Medicine
FVC	forced vital capacity
GMC	General Medical Council
HAART	highly active antiretroviral therapy
HACCP	hazard analysis and critical control point
HAVS	hand arm vibration syndrome
HDI	hexamethylene diisocyanate
HGV	heavy goods vehicle
HSE	Health and Safety Executive
IIDB	Industrial Injuries Disablement Benefit
LTOT	Long-term oxygen therapy
MAC	manual handling assessment chart
NICE	National Institute for Health and Care Excellence
OH	Occupational Health
PCB	polychlorinated biphenyl
PPE	personal protective equipment
RIDDOR	Reporting of Injuries, Diseases and Dangerous Occurrences Regulations
SEQOHS	Safe, Effective, Quality, Occupational Health Service
TB	tuberculosis
TIA	transient ischaemic attack
TTMA	trans,trans-muconic acid
ULD	upper limb disorder
VDU	visual display unit
VTEC	verotoxin-producing *Escherichia coli*
WEL	workplace exposure limit
WRAP	Wellbeing Recovery Action Plan

Introduction to the exam

Style

The diploma examination (DOccMed) is divided into two parts:

- a written paper with a style of questioning that requires you to provide the 'best possible fit' answer to the question; this means that in some cases there may be more than one possible answer, but the correct answer will be the one which is the most appropriate; for example, the action that should be done as the first line or the gold standard response.
- a portfolio submission and oral assessment on the subject of your portfolio.

You can take both parts in the same sitting. I found this to be ideal, because I was already revising for the written exam and the oral examination questions are along similar lines. However, many people take the exams at separate sittings and you have up to five years between the portfolio/oral examination and the written exam. A maximum of six attempts at the exams can be made.

The written exam

The written exam must be completed in 90 minutes. The number of questions varies per sitting but is usually approximately 70 and the Faculty of Occupational Medicine (FOM) states that the minimum number will be 50. The pass mark also varies, but it is typically around 75%, with the actual level dependent on the difficulty of the paper. Very importantly, the exam is not negatively marked and so it is worth hazarding a guess if you are not sure of the answer! Please be aware that the FOM sometimes trials new questions in the exam.

Questions may be asked on any part of the core syllabus and all pertain to occupational health practice in the UK and the application of UK laws.

You will be provided with a machine-readable sheet on which to record your answers. Candidates are required to record their answer by blacking out the box at the corresponding number for that statement on the answer sheet with a pencil. There is no need for a calculator but an eraser is a useful tool! **Only one answer per question may be chosen**.

The portfolio and oral assessment

The portfolio consists of two pieces of written work, with a combined word count of between 1500 and 2000. The first piece of work is based on a visit, assessment and analysis of a workplace by the candidate – this can be anything from an office to a hairdressing salon. The second piece of work is a clinical case (this must be a case seen and assessed by you) written from an occupational health perspective; for example, a person with carpal tunnel syndrome affecting their ability to work as a typist.

The portfolio is not written under exam conditions – you can do this in your own time. It is useful to get somebody working in occupational health to read it over before you submit it! The portfolio must obviously be submitted before the exam deadline. Two occupational health experts will assess your portfolio and then ask you questions related solely to your portfolio. So, for example, if your workplace assessment is based on a glue factory they will not ask you about the laws surrounding working with asbestos! The oral examination should be no longer than half an hour.

You will be marked on:
- your written and oral communication skills
- presentation – marks may be deducted for poor presentation
- content – you must demonstrate that you understand the principles of occupational health medicine in the UK and can apply them in practice.

The pass mark for the portfolio and oral examination is 50%.

Diploma course

It is a requirement of the diploma that you complete an FOM-approved course before sitting the exams. These can be completed at numerous centres.

Further information

The syllabus for the diploma and the portfolio template can be found on the Faculty of Occupational Medicine website (www.fom.ac.uk), in addition to a few example questions.

CHAPTER 1
Ethics and law

Which of the following conditions is specifically not considered to be a disability under the Equality Act 2010?

a) Liver cirrhosis
b) Alcoholism
c) Disfigurement
d) Anxiety
e) Diabetes

QUESTION 2: EQUALITY ACT 2010

Which of the following conditions is specifically not considered to be a disability under the Equality Act 2010?

a) Obesity
b) Depression
c) Melanoma
d) Chronic fatigue syndrome
e) Asthma

QUESTION 3: REASONABLE ADJUSTMENTS

Under the Equality Act 2010, an employer has a duty to provide reasonable adjustments. Which of the following statements is true?

a) The failure to provide reasonable adjustments can be justified
b) This applies to those employees who care for a disabled person
c) Reasonable adjustments should be provided regardless of cost
d) Employers must disregard all disability-related sickness absence
e) Employers can treat a disabled employee more favourably than others

QUESTION 4: DISPLAY SCREEN EQUIPMENT (DSE)

Regarding working with DSE and DSE Regulations 1992, which of the following statements is true?

a) By law 15-minute breaks must be taken every 4 hours
b) Pregnant women are legally required to work reduced hours at a computer
c) A work laptop must undergo DSE assessment
d) Work placement students are covered by the DSE Regulations
e) They apply to every employee who uses a computer in the workplace

QUESTION 5: PERSONAL PROTECTIVE EQUIPMENT (PPE) REGULATIONS

Which of the following is stated in the PPE Regulations 1992?

a) PPE should be provided when risks cannot be controlled any other way
b) PPE should be CE marked
c) PPE should be risk assessed so that it is appropriate for individuals
d) PPE should be free of charge
e) All of the above

QUESTION 6: WORKPLACE REGULATIONS

Which of the following is not covered under the Workplace (Health, Safety and Welfare) Regulations 1992?

a) Toileting facilities
b) Breastfeeding facilities
c) Minimum room sizes
d) Workplace road surfaces
e) None of the above

QUESTION 7: WORKPLACE REGULATIONS

Which of the following workplaces are not covered under the Workplace (Health, Safety and Welfare) Regulations 1992?

a) Hospitals
b) Shipyards
c) Trading floors
d) Children's nurseries
e) Arboretums

QUESTION 8: THE 'SIX PACK'

Which of the following regulations is not part of the 'Six Pack' regulations?

a) Provision and Use of Work Equipment Regulations 1998
b) Reporting of Injuries, Diseases and Dangerous Occurrences Regulations 1995
c) Management of Health and Safety at Work Regulations 1999
d) Personal Protective Equipment Regulations 2002
e) Workplace (Health, Safety and Welfare) Regulations 1992

QUESTION 9: CONSENT

Regarding consent, which of the following statements is true?

a) Expressed consent is needed for reports to be sent to an employer
b) Informed consent is not needed to take part in health surveillance
c) When the employee requests to see the occupational health report before the employer this should always be done
d) Implied consent is not appropriate for phlebotomy
e) Consent cannot be withdrawn

QUESTION 10: CONTROL OF SUBSTANCES HAZARDOUS TO HEALTH (COSHH) 2002

Which of the following is not covered under COSHH 2002?

a) *Legionella pneumophilia*
b) Poly aromatic hydrocarbons
c) Lead
d) Flour
e) Silver

QUESTION 11: COSHH 2002

What factors would make an organization re-evaluate their controls?

a) Accidents
b) Feedback
c) Legislation
d) Redundancy
e) All of the above

QUESTION 12: DATA PROTECTION ACT 1998

Which of the following is incorrect with regard to the Data Protection Act 1998?

a) Clinicians have 40 days in which to supply medical records
b) Clinicians can charge for access to medical records by the individual
c) Clinicians cannot withhold access to medical records
d) Medical records cannot be kept in the boot of a car
e) All of the above

QUESTION 13: DISABILITY DISCRIMINATION

In which year was the Disability Discrimination Act 1995 superseded?

a) 1995
b) 2000
c) 2002
d) 2010
e) 2015

QUESTION 14: DSE REGULATIONS 1992

Which of the following is not part of the Health and Safety (DSE) Regulations 1992?

a) Vision screening is mandatory
b) Risk assessments must be carried out on the employee's workstation when using a VDU (visual display unit)
c) A VDU user is a person who uses a VDU for more than one hour a day, or who relies on a VDU for work
d) A calculator is not a VDU under the above regulations
e) An adjustable chair is included as one of the minimum requirements for a VDU user under the above regulations

QUESTION 15: THE HEALTH AND SAFETY AT WORK ACT (HASAWA) 1974

Which of the following is not covered under HASAWA 1974?

a) Employees have a need to comply with statutory health and safety measures enforced by the employer
b) Manufacturers have a duty to provide information about their product
c) Specialists who provide advice are liable if the advice causes harm
d) Controllers of premises have a duty to ensure that they are well maintained
e) None of the above

QUESTION 16: FIRST AID

Which of the following is correct?

a) First aiders do not need certification
b) First aiders must have refresher training every 2 years
c) An accident book is a legal requirement
d) There is no specific regulation regarding first aid at work
e) None of the above

QUESTION 17: RIDDOR

Which of the following is not a reportable disease under RIDDOR 2013 (Reporting of Injuries, Diseases and Dangerous Occurrences Regulations)?

a) Severe arm cramp
b) Carpal tunnel
c) Asthma
d) Hand arm vibration syndrome (HAVS)
e) None of the above

QUESTION 18: NOISE REGULATIONS

At what level does an employer need to make an area a hearing protection zone?

a) 80 decibels
b) 82 decibels
c) 85 decibels
d) 87 decibels
e) 112 decibels

QUESTION 19: DISABILITY

Which of the following is part of the legal definition of disability?

a) Must last 6 consecutive months or more
b) Must last 6 weeks or more
c) Must last 12 weeks or more
d) Must last 12 consecutive weeks or more
e) Must last 12 months or more

QUESTION 20: HASAWA 1974

Which section of HASAWA 1974 does the following paragraph apply to?

'[Employers must] SO FAR AS IS REASONABLY PRACTICABLE ensure contractors are not exposed to risks to their health and safety...'

a) Section 2
b) Section 3
c) Section 4
d) Section 6
e) None of the above

QUESTION 21: MEDICAL RECORDS

Mr Smith, a radiologist, wants to see his occupational health reports. Which of the following statements is true?

a) Clinicians have 30 days in which to supply medical records
b) It is not recommended to charge for access to reports
c) Access to medical reports cannot be withheld
d) All records relating to the Ionizing Radiation Regulations 1999 must be kept for 30 years by law
e) He must make this request in writing

QUESTION 22: STATUTES

The principle of 'so far as is reasonably possible' is outlined in which of the following statutes?

a) The Management of Health and Safety Regulations 1999
b) Workplace (Health, Safety and Welfare) Regulations 1992
c) The Health and Safety at Work Act 1974
d) The Provision and Use of Work Equipment Regulations 1992
e) All of the above

QUESTION 23: RIDDOR

Which of the following is reportable under RIDDOR 2013?

a) A fall resulting in eight stitches in the Accident and Emergency Department
b) A fall resulting in a brief loss of consciousness
c) A fall resulting in a thumb dislocation
d) A fall resulting in a fracture of the index finger
e) A fall resulting in back pain leading to four days' absence from work

QUESTION 24: DISABILITY

Which of the following is true regarding disability?

a) Must last 12 consecutive months or more
b) If medication resolves the employee's symptoms then the employee cannot be classified as disabled
c) Cannot be retrospectively based
d) Must be expected to last 12 months or more
e) If the employee has access to aids that make them more productive than an able-bodied person then they can no longer be classed as disabled

QUESTION 25: CONFIDENTIALITY

Regarding confidentiality – which of the following is incorrect?

a) Confidentiality is not absolute
b) Physicians must consult with a defence union before breaking confidentiality
c) Breaking confidentiality is a last resort
d) In the interest of public safety confidentiality can be broken
e) A coroner's court can request confidential information

QUESTION 26: CONSENT

Regarding occupational health confidentiality – in which scenario can the information be released without expressed consent, assuming all efforts have been made to obtain consent?

a) Releasing information regarding a new case of streptococcal pneumonia to Public Health England
b) Releasing the details of a Group 1 driver with poorly controlled migraines who continues to drive against medical advice to the DVLA (Driver and Vehicle Licensing Agency)
c) Releasing any information once a person has died
d) Releasing information to the coroner in the case of a fatal accident at work
e) Releasing the CD4 count of a mechanic with HIV to employers

QUESTION 27: COSHH 2002

Legally, how long must records relating to COSHH 2002 be kept for?

a) 10 years
b) 20 years
c) 40 years
d) 80 years
e) 100 years

QUESTION 28: EQUALITY ACT 2010

You are reviewing your employer's disability policy. Which of the following is not covered by the Equality Act 2010?

a) Gender reassignment
b) Marital status
c) Social class
d) Maternity
e) Religious beliefs

QUESTION 29: ETHICS

Which of the following is not correct?

a) Expressed consent is needed for reports to be sent to an employer
b) Informed consent is needed to take part in health surveillance
c) When the employee requests to see the occupational health report before the employer this should always be done
d) Implied consent is appropriate for phlebotomy
e) None of the above

QUESTION 30: REASONABLE ADJUSTMENTS

A call centre worker is suffering with depression resulting in an inability to concentrate at work. She has only seen her GP. Which of the following statements is correct?

a) If her employer raises a disciplinary against her symptoms this is direct discrimination
b) She is entitled to reasonable adjustments
c) Depression is unlikely to be classed as a disability
d) Employers should ask whether her decreased productivity is due to ill health
e) None of the above

QUESTION 31: REASONABLE ADJUSTMENTS

Which of the following is not classed as a reasonable adjustment?

a) Text to speech software
b) Sign language interpreter
c) Wheelchair
d) Penguin mouse
e) None of the above

QUESTION 32: COSHH 2002

Which of the following is incorrect?

a) COSHH only applies if there is a workplace exposure limit
b) Control measures should be proportionate to risk
c) Employees should undertake training in the risks of the work involved
d) PPE should only be used as a last resort
e) Control measures should not increase other safety risks

QUESTION 33: GOOD OCCUPATIONAL HEALTH PRACTICE

Which of the following is part of the Faculty of Occupational Medicine's (FOM) good occupational health practice guidelines?

a) Revalidation
b) Audit
c) Education of others
d) Transfer of services
e) All of the above

QUESTION 34: VIBRATION REGULATIONS

Under the Control of Vibration at Work Regulations 2005, for hand arm vibration, which is the level of vibration at which action needs to be taken to reduce exposure?

a) 1.5 m/s^2 A(8)
b) 2.0 m/s^2 A(8)
c) 2.5 m/s^2 A(8)
d) 5.0 m/s^2 A(8)
e) None of the above

QUESTION 35: COSHH 2002

Regarding working with dust, which of the following statements is correct?

a) Some masks require the wearer to be clean shaven
b) Dry sweeping is better than wet cleaning
c) When working outside, masks are generally not needed
d) Quick tasks do not require masks
e) Members of the public are at risk of new lung disease during street works

QUESTION 36: LAW

Which of the following does not have specific statutory requirements for health surveillance?

a) Noise
b) Compressed air
c) Vibration
d) Working at heights
e) Radiation

ANSWERS to Ethics and law questions

QUESTION 1: EQUALITY ACT 2010

Which of the following conditions is specifically not considered to be a disability under the Equality Act 2010?

The answer is: b) Alcoholism

- Alcoholism and drug addictions are not considered to be disabling conditions under the Equality Act 2010.
- However, the sequelae of alcohol addiction can be considered disabling if they fulfil the required criteria.
- Severe disfigurement (not including piercings and tattoos) can be considered disabling.

QUESTION 2: EQUALITY ACT 2010

Which of the following conditions is specifically not considered to be a disability under the Equality Act 2010?

The answer is: a) Obesity

A 2014 European Court case found that there is no law classifying obesity as a disability.

However, the sequelae of obesity could result in a person being disabled.

QUESTION 3: REASONABLE ADJUSTMENTS

Under the Equality Act 2010, an employer has a duty to provide reasonable adjustments. Which of the following statements is true?

The answer is: e) Employers can treat a disabled employee more favourably than others

The Equality Act 2010 requires 'reasonable adjustments' to be made to allow disabled employees to work:

- These range from auxiliary aids to disabled parking spaces.
- These must be related to the job and only apply to the employee and not others.
- This also means that employers can treat disabled employees or potential employees more favourably to make up for their substantial disadvantage.
- Failure to provide reasonable adjustments cannot be justified in court, but the reasonable adjustment can be based on cost, effectiveness and other criteria.

QUESTION 4: DISPLAY SCREEN EQUIPMENT

Regarding working with DSE and DSE Regulations 1992, which of the following statements is true?

The answer is: c) A work laptop must undergo DSE assessment

- DSE Regulations do not specify the number or length of breaks; they only specify that DSE users should take regular breaks.
- DSE Regulations apply to portable equipment.
- DSE does not emit radiation.
- The DSE Regulations do not cover students or those who use DSE for less than one hour a day.

QUESTION 5: PPE REGULATIONS

Which of the following is stated in the PPE Regulations 1992?

The answer is: e) All of the above

The PPE Regulations 1992 state that PPE should be supplied at work by the employer when risks cannot be controlled any other way. When they can be controlled in another way, they should be, because PPE is the last and least effective form of control.

- PPE should be free of charge.
- PPE should be CE marked, which means it complies with the European basic safety standards.
- PPE should be risk assessed for suitability and compatibility.
- PPE must be stored and maintained safely so there must be appropriate systems for reporting loss and damage.

- Training and information should be provided on the use of PPE and also the risks that the employees are faced with.
- PPE includes all that is worn or held to minimize risks. This includes risks from weather.

QUESTION 6: WORKPLACE REGULATIONS

Which of the following is not covered under the Workplace (Health, Safety and Welfare) Regulations 1992?

The answer is: e) None of the above

The Workplace (Health, Safety and Welfare) Regulations 1992 cover a wide range of basic health, safety and welfare issues and apply to most workplaces.

QUESTION 7: WORKPLACE REGULATIONS

Which of the following workplaces are not covered under the Workplace (Health, Safety and Welfare) Regulations 1992?

The answer is: b) Shipyards

The Workplace (Health, Safety and Welfare) Regulations 1992 do not cover construction workplaces and shipyards.

QUESTION 8: THE 'SIX PACK'

Which of the following regulations is not part of the 'Six Pack' regulations?

The answer is: b) Reporting of Injuries, Diseases and Dangerous Occurrences Regulations 1995

'Six Pack' regulations are prescriptive regulations giving details on how to carry out the Health and Safety at Work Act 1974. They include the following:
- Management of Health and Safety at Work Regulations 1999.
- Personal Protective Equipment Regulations 2002.
- Workplace (Health, Safety and Welfare) Regulations 1992.
- The Provision and Use of Work Equipment Regulations 1998.
- Health and Safety (Display Screen Equipment) Regulations 1992.
- Manual Handling Operations Regulations 1992.

QUESTION 9: CONSENT

Regarding consent, which of the following statements is true?

The answer is: a) Expressed consent is needed for reports to be sent to an employer

It is not always appropriate for the employee to see the report before the employer, even when the employee requests this. These instances would include the following:
- The report contains material that will be considered harmful to the employee's health.
- The report contains information about a third party who has not consented to its release.

Expressed consent is needed:
- From the employer to get someone seen by the occupational health team.
- From the employer for the occupational health physician to allow consultation.
- For the report to be sent to the employer.
- To gain access to specialist medical reports and GP medical reports from the employee. The Access to Medical Reports Act 1988 gives the patient the right to see medical reports prepared by a doctor responsible for their care for employment and insurance purposes.

It is good practice to offer the patient the chance to see the report before the employer, or at the same time as the employer.

QUESTION 10: COSHH 2002

Which of the following is not covered under COSHH 2002?

The answer is: c) Lead

- COSHH covers substances that are hazardous to health. Substances can take many forms including: chemicals, products containing chemicals, fumes, dusts and germs that cause disease.
- COSHH does not cover lead, asbestos or radiation because these have their own specific regulations.
- *Legionella pneumophilia* causes legionnaires' disease, which is an occupational disease associated with those who work with hot and cold water systems.

QUESTION 11: COSHH 2002

What factors would make an organization re-evaluate their controls?

The answer is: e) All of the above

Controls should be re-evaluated and new risk assessments done routinely.

Other reasons to instigate a re-evaluation include:
- New legislation
- New information from the manufacturer
- Complaints
- Accidents.

QUESTION 12: DATA PROTECTION ACT 1998

Which of the following is incorrect with regard to the Data Protection Act 1998?

The answer is: c) Clinicians cannot withhold access to medical records

The **Data Protection Act** covers the storage, collection and access to medical records – not to be confused with the **Access to Medical Records Act 1988**. It states that:
- The basic principles of data protection include health-related information – which should be stored for as long as is necessary – and outline the terms of 40 years for COSHH regulations and 50 years for the ionizing radiation regulations, but they do not stipulate a time period for normal occupational health records.
- Data should be kept secure – but it does stipulate that records can be kept in the boot of a car if necessary, but not overnight, and in normal circumstances they should be kept in a locked filing cabinet or as encrypted data.
- Information obtained should be lawful and for a specific purpose – it should be accurate, kept up to date, and the minimum information needed should be recorded.

Under this Act:
- Clinicians are given 40 days to supply the relevant information and the individual has to give written notice of request.
- Clinicians can withhold access to records if the records include:
  - Information about a third party who has not consented for disclosure.
  - Information that might cause serious harm to the patient and/or others.

QUESTION 13: DISABILITY DISCRIMINATION

In which year was the Disability Discrimination Act 1995 superseded?

The answer is: d) 2010

The Disability Discrimination Act (DDA) was replaced by The Equality Act 2010 in the UK, except Northern Ireland, where the DDA still applies.

QUESTION 14: DSE REGULATIONS 1992

Which of the following is not part of the Health and Safety (DSE) Regulations 1992?

The answer is: a) Vision screening is mandatory

The Health and Safety (DSE) 1992 Regulations in short state that:
- **Risk assessments** – must be carried out on the employee's workstation if they are a VDU user – this includes the equipment, the workspace (including the furniture) and the environment.
- **Eye testing** – must be provided by the employer on request. The employer must cover the expense of spectacles for employees who require it for using display screen equipment only.
- **Regular breaks** – must be taken when using display screen equipment.
- **Workstations** – ensure they meet the minimum requirements, including adjustable chairs and that the keyboard can be tilted to avoid fatigue of the hands and arms.
- **VDUs** – ensure appropriate information is provided to the employee about VDUs to minimize their risk.

QUESTION 15: HASAWA 1974

Which of the following is not covered under HASAWA 1974?

The answer is: e) None of the above

The Health and Safety at Work Act 1974 outlines the duties of employers, employees, manufacturers, importers and controllers of premises amongst others, to ensure so far as is reasonably practicable the health and safety of workers. Employers have a duty of care to their employees and third parties and have to ensure that:
- The premises are well maintained.
- Substances are handled with due care.

- Information and training is provided to those on the premises to reduce risk.
- PPE needs to be provided free of charge.
- Employees in turn have to not undertake actions that will harm themselves or fellow employees, and have to undertake the statutory requirements to reduce health and safety risks when enforced by the employer.
- Manufacturers have to ensure that their products are made safely, information is provided for their safe use, and maintenance and testing is provided when need be.
- Controllers of premises have to ensure that their premises are kept safe.
- Employers also have to provide information on risks to third parties entering the premises or working on the premises.

QUESTION 16: FIRST AID

Which of the following is correct?

The answer is: c) An accident book is a legal requirement

Under the **First Aid at Work Regulations 1981**, first aiders must be certified and have refresher training every 3 years. An accident book and first aid box suitable to the risks are legal requirements under the regulations.

QUESTION 17: RIDDOR

Which of the following is not a reportable disease under RIDDOR 2013?

The answer is: e) None of the above

The RIDDOR regulations state what occupational diseases, injuries and near-misses need to be reported and within what timescale. There are eight occupational diseases that need to be reported:
- HAVS
- Severe arm cramp
- Carpal tunnel
- Occupational asthma
- Occupational dermatitis
- Occupational cancers
- Diseases attributable to biological agents
- Tendonitis.

QUESTION 18: NOISE REGULATONS

At what level does an employer need to make an area a hearing protection zone?

The answer is: c) 85 decibels

Under the Noise Regulations 2005:
- **80 decibels** is the lower exposure action value. At this level, health surveillance must be provided and personal protective equipment must be provided if asked for by the employee.
- **85 decibels** is the upper exposure action value. At this level, hearing protection must be worn, the area must be designated a hearing protection zone and, again, health surveillance must be undertaken.
- **87 decibels** is the upper limit value. Employees must not be exposed to noise above this level. This may include stopping work, and sound pressure limits: the lower exposure action value for sound pressure limits is 112 Pa; the upper exposure action value is 140 Pa; and the exposure limit value is 200 Pa.

QUESTION 19: DISABILITY

Which of the following is part of the legal definition of disability?

The answer is: e) Must last 12 months or more

To qualify as having a disability (with the exception of conditions that automatically qualify) a person must have a condition that:
- Is mental or physical.
- Has a substantial impact on ADL (activities of daily living).
- Must last 12 months or more (these do not have to be consecutive) OR be expected to last 12 months or more.
- This must be based on the natural history of the disease, irrespective of whether the patient is on medication or not.

QUESTION 20: HASAWA 1974

Which section of HASAWA 1974 does the following paragraph apply to:
'[Employers must] SO FAR AS IS REASONABLY PRACTICABLE ensure contractors are not exposed to risks to their health and safety...'

The answer is: b) Section 3

Regarding the Health and Safety at Work Act 1974 the duties of employers and employees to one another are outlined.

It is important to know the main segments:
- Section 2: outlines duties of employers to employees.
- Section 3: outlines duties to third parties (including contractors).
- Section 6: duties of manufacturers, importers and suppliers.
- Section 7: duties of employees.

QUESTION 21: MEDICAL RECORDS

Mr Smith, a radiologist, wants to see his occupational health reports. Which of the following statements is true?

The answer is: e) He must make this request in writing

Under **The Data Protection Act 1998**:
- Clinicians are given 40 days to supply the relevant information and the individual has to give written notice of request.
- Clinicians can withhold access to records if the records include:
  - Information about a third party who has not consented for disclosure.
  - Information that might cause serious harm to the patient and/or others.

QUESTION 22: STATUTES

The principle of 'so far as is reasonably possible' is outlined in which of the following statutes?

The answer is: c) The Health and Safety at Work Act 1974

The table below outlines some of the main statutory regulations that you need to know about.

STATUTES	OUTLINE OF MAIN PRINCIPLES
Health and Safety at Work Act 1974	The risk to health and safety at work should be reduced so far as is reasonably possible. This Act outlines the duties of the employers towards the employee and third parties, including the public; the duties of the controllers of the premises; the duties of the employees; and the duties of those who manufacture, sell and import equipment, to ensure that the risk to health and safety is reduced so far as is reasonably practicable.
Workplace (Health, Safety and Welfare) Regulations 1992	These outline the minimum requirements for the workplace, including emergency lighting, temperature, size, hygiene and requirements for rest rooms and toilet facilities.
COSHH 2002	The need for risk assessment when working with chemicals and biological agents, and for health surveillance.
RIDDOR 2013	The Reporting of Injuries, Diseases and Dangerous Occurrences Regulations outline the need to report certain injuries, diseases and near-misses and set out the required time in which do so. They also set out the need to report injuries that result in over 7 days' absence from work.

QUESTION 23: RIDDOR

Which of the following is reportable under RIDDOR 2013?

The answer is: b) A fall resulting in a brief loss of consciousness

The RIDDOR regulations state what occupational diseases, injuries and near-misses need to be reported and within what timescale.

Under RIDDOR the following need to be reported:
- Deaths at work.
- Any injuries requiring hospitalization or involving loss of consciousness.
- Fractures of the long bones.
- Loss of sight.
- Injuries or work-related illnesses resulting in over 7 days' absence from work.

Reporting can be done to the HSE (Health and Safety Executive) online or via the telephone.

QUESTION 24: DISABILITY

Which of the following is true regarding disability?

The answer is: d) Must be expected to last 12 months or more

To the finer detail of qualifying as having a disability (with the exception of conditions that automatically qualify) in the legal sense:

- Must last 12 months or more (these do not have to be consecutive) OR be expected to last 12 months or more – so it can be labelled as having a disability at the beginning of the course of the disease.
- This must be based on the natural history of the disease, irrespective of whether the patient is on medication or not.
- This is regardless of how productive an individual is with or without adjustments/aids.
- This can be retrospectively based, so if a person has overcome the illness/problem that made them disadvantaged then they still can be classed as disabled. This is important in cases of discrimination. However, it can only be retrospective if ALL the criteria are met AND it is since the legislation came into effect (2010).

QUESTION 25: CONFIDENTIALITY

Regarding confidentiality – which of the following is incorrect?

The answer is: b) Physicians must consult with a defence union before breaking confidentiality

It is advisable that a physician consults with their defence union before breaking confidentiality, but this is not a mandatory requirement.

Confidentiality is never absolute and patients must be informed that there may be times when their confidential information may be released without their consent. However, in practice all efforts must be made to allow the patient to give consent for the information to be released or to release the information themselves.

Confidentiality can be broken in the following circumstances:

- In the interest of public safety.
- If ordered by a court.
- If it is in the public's interest.
- If it is required by law/statute.

QUESTION 26: CONSENT

Regarding occupational health confidentiality – in which scenario can the information be released without expressed consent, assuming all efforts have been made to obtain consent?

The answer is: d) Releasing information to the coroner in the case of a fatal accident at work

Confidentiality can be broken in the following circumstances:
- In the interest of public safety.
- If ordered by a court.
- If it is in the public's interest.

This includes notifiable diseases; information regarding those unfit to drive in accordance with DVLA guidance; and cases where non-disclosure will put others at risk of serious harm including the prevention of serious crime.

In the case of the deceased, your duty of confidentiality continues after death, but information should be released to help in the case of inquests and in the coroner's court.

In all cases the principles of data protection apply; the information released should be:
- To a minimum needed
- Accurate
- Relevant
- To as few people as possible.

QUESTION 27: COSHH 2002

Legally, how long must records relating to COSHH 2002 be kept for?

The answer is: c) 40 years

General information should be stored for as long as necessary, but specifically:
- 40 years for information regarding COSHH Regulations.
- 50 years for the information related to Ionizing Radiation Regulations.

QUESTION 28: EQUALITY ACT 2010

You are reviewing your employer's disability policy. Which of the following is not covered by the Equality Act 2010?

The answer is: c) Social class

Under the Equality Act 2010, the following characteristics are protected from discrimination:
- **Age**
- **Sex**
- **Race**
- **Religion or beliefs**
- **Pregnancy or maternity**
- **Marital/civil partnership status**
- **Gender reassignment**
- **Sexual orientation.**

QUESTION 29: ETHICS

Which of the following is not correct?

The answer is: c) When the employee requests to see the occupational health report before the employer this should always be done

Expressed consent is needed:
- From the employer to get someone seen by the occupational health team.
- From the employer for the occupational health physician to allow consultation.
- For the report to be sent to the employer.
- To gain access to specialist medical reports and GP medical reports from the employee.
- It is good practice to offer the patient the chance to see the report before the employer or at the same time as the employer.

Occupational health reports undergo the principle of no surprises, that is, the employee should be absolutely clear about what process they are engaging in and also what information will be reported about them to a third party.

Informed consent, with regard to health surveillance, involves the following:
- An explanation about why health surveillance is being undertaken.
- How it will be undertaken.

- What information will be taken.
- Who will have access to that information.
- How it will be stored.
- What action will be taken if there is a positive result.

QUESTION 30: REASONABLE ADJUSTMENTS

A call centre worker is suffering with depression resulting in an inability to concentrate at work. She has only seen her GP. Which of the following statements is correct?

The answer is: d) Employers should ask whether her decreased productivity is due to ill health

An employer only has to provide reasonable adjustments if they know, or could reasonably be expected to know that the employee has a disability.

The employer must, however, do all that they reasonably can to find out whether this is the case.

QUESTION 31: REASONABLE ADJUSTMENTS

Which of the following is not classed as a reasonable adjustment?

The answer is: c) Wheelchair

An employer only has to provide reasonable adjustments to someone with a disability if it is connected to the job; there is no requirement to provide or modify equipment relating to personal needs.

QUESTION 32: COSHH 2002

Which of the following is incorrect?

The answer is: a) COSHH only applies if there is a workplace exposure limit

Under COSHH regulations, eight principles apply regardless of whether a substance has a workplace exposure limit. These are:
- Design and operate processes and activities to minimize spread of substances hazardous to health.
- Take into account all relevant routes of exposure.

- Control exposure by measures that are proportionate to the health risk.
- Choose the most effective and reliable control options.
- Where adequate control of exposure cannot be achieved by other means, provide, in combination with other control measures, suitable personal protective equipment.
- Check and review regularly all elements of control measures.
- Inform and train all employees on the hazards and risks from the substances with which they work.
- Ensure that the introduction of control measures does not increase the overall risk to health and safety.

QUESTION 33: GOOD OCCUPATIONAL HEALTH PRACTICE

Which of the following is part of the FOM's good occupational health practice guidelines?

The answer is: e) All of the above

Included in the guidance:
- Good clinical care including providing good clinical care and supporting self-care.
- Raising concerns about patient safety.
- Maintaining good medical practice including keeping up to date and improving practice; teaching and training; and appraising and assessing.
- Maintaining the doctor–patient partnership including good communication, consent, and confidentiality.
- Ending your professional relationship including taking up and ending appointments.
- Probity, integrity and honesty.

QUESTION 34: VIBRATION REGULATIONS

Under the **Control of Vibration at Work Regulations 2005**, for hand arm vibration, which is the level of vibration at which action needs to be taken to reduce exposure?

The answer is: c) 2.5 m/s² A(8)

The Control of Vibration at Work Regulations 2005:
- Exposure action values (EAVs) indicate the level of vibration at which action must be taken to reduce exposure.
- Exposure limit values (ELVs) set the maximum level of vibration that should not be exceeded in any single day.

Both types of value are calculated as the average exposure experienced over an eight-hour period.

For hand arm vibration:
- The exposure action value is 2.5 m/s^2 A(8).
- The exposure limit value is 5.0 m/s^2 A(8).

For whole body vibration:
- The exposure action value is 0.5 m/s^2 A(8).
- The exposure limit value is 1.15 m/s^2 A(8).

QUESTION 35: COSHH 2002

Regarding working with dust, which of the following statements is correct?

The answer is: a) Some masks require the wearer to be clean shaven

- Tight fit respirators require a face fit and the wearer to be clean shaven for the mask to be fitted properly.
- Wet cleaning is where the dust is wetted before it is cleaned away and is a reasonable method of removing dust; sweeping it when it is dry means that more of it is swept into the air.
- The risk of lung disease when working with dust is generally from the cumulative effects, so over time, even for quick tasks or when working outside (where wind may carry the dust away), this means that the risk is not removed. For this reason also, members of the public are generally not exposed for long enough periods of time for lung disease to occur (although exposure for any length of time may trigger already diagnosed lung disease, for example, asthma).

QUESTION 36: LAW

Which of the following does not have specific statutory requirements for health surveillance?

The answer is: d) Working at heights

There are specific regulations for:
- Noise
- Lead
- Asbestos
- Diving
- Working with compressed air
- Radiation
- Vibration.

CHAPTER 2
Effects of work on health

You see a 60-year-old carpenter who has worked with asbestos in the past. He has had an X-ray that has been reported as showing pleural plaques. Which of the following is incorrect?

a) They are pathognomic of asbestos exposure
b) It does not qualify for IIDB (Industrial Injuries Disablement Benefit)
c) He can sue his employer for asbestos exposure
d) Pleural plaques are benign
e) Pleural plaques affect the visceral pleura

QUESTION 2: BLOOD-BORNE VIRUS

A student nurse comes to an NHS clinic after a needle-stick injury. She has not been vaccinated against hepatitis B. She is very worried about her risk of contracting a blood-borne virus. Her approximate risk is...

a) 1 in 3
b) 1 in 30
c) 1 in 300
d) 1 in 3000
e) 1 in 3 million

QUESTION 3: DERMATITIS

Ms Pryor is setting up a hairdressing business. She wants advice on how to control the risk of dermatitis. Which of the following measures is useful for her?

a) Wet work policy
b) Visual inspection
c) Questionnaires
d) Prompt clean-up of spillages
e) All of the above

QUESTION 4: DIABETES

Diabetic lorry drivers…

a) Automatically qualify as disabled under the Equality Act 2010
b) Cannot work in safety-critical roles due to the risk of hypos
c) On insulin need a two-yearly medical examination
d) On metformin must monitor their blood glucose at least twice a day
e) Must notify the DVLA (Driver and Vehicle Licensing Agency) regardless of whether or not they are on treatment

QUESTION 5: EPILEPSY

Mr Smith has well-controlled epilepsy. He has not had a seizure in 12 years. He has not told his employers about his condition. Which of the following statements is true?

a) He is under a legal obligation to disclose his condition to his employers
b) Potential employers are never allowed to enquire about his health conditions before offering him a job
c) If his epilepsy interferes with his ability to do his job safely then his employers may dismiss him
d) He cannot hold a Group 2 driving licence
e) He can join the army

QUESTION 6: EPILEPSY

You see a man diagnosed with epilepsy who wants to go back to work as an HGV (heavy goods vehicle) driver. He has been seizure-free for a number of years. How many years must he be seizure-free before he can have a Group 2 licence?

a) 3
b) 5
c) 9
d) 10
e) 12

QUESTION 7: OCCUPATIONAL DISEASES

Which of the following diseases is associated with coal mining?

a) Rheumatoid arthritis
b) Bladder cancer
c) Asthma
d) Renal failure
e) Angiosarcoma

QUESTION 8: HAND ARM VIBRATION SYNDROME (HAVS)

You see a 35-year-old ship builder who is having difficulty picking up small objects; you suspect he has HAVS. Which of the following is correct?

a) Smoking worsens HAVS
b) Symptoms do not occur in hot weather
c) Appropriate employee clothing can prevent HAVS
d) Amlodipine is useful in the management of HAVS
e) Tingling is a late sign

QUESTION 9: HEARING

You discover that a patient in a printing factory has suffered from noise-induced hearing loss. Which of the following statements is true?

a) Employers have no legal duty to move employees against their wishes
b) Caucasians are genetically susceptible to noise-induced hearing loss
c) Those in the printing industry are at risk of conductive hearing loss
d) Consent is not needed to release personal information to the Health and Safety Executive (HSE)
e) Workers do not need to be informed of anonymized surveillance data being released

QUESTION 10: HEARING

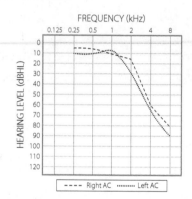

Whilst undertaking hearing surveillance of factory workers you come across this audiogram of an employee. Which of the following statements is correct?

a) This patient has bilateral noise-induced hearing loss
b) A full history and examination should be undertaken to determine the cause of hearing loss
c) All doctors working in occupational health can undertake hearing surveillance
d) Hearing surveillance is a legal requirement in all factories
e) Ear plugs are the best form of control where there is a risk of noise-induced hearing loss

QUESTION 11: MENTAL HEALTH

You see a fireman who has been struggling at work recently. You think that he has a diagnosis of depression. Which of the following statements is correct?

a) Presenteeism is not an issue in mental health illness
b) You should start him on sertraline as per NICE guidance
c) The Boorman Report recommends that management in the fire service should be trained in recognizing mental health problems
d) Night shift work may not be advisable in his case
e) He should be advised not to work in the fire department due to the stressful nature of the job

QUESTION 12: OCCUPATIONAL ASTHMA

You undertake screening in a bakery in which a case of occupational asthma has been diagnosed. You see a gentleman who has a wheeze that only occurs at work. Which of the following statements is true?

a) A respiratory mask will help alleviate his condition
b) Legally his employer should relocate him
c) This case falls under the Equality Act 2010
d) Employers must make sure that the workplace exposure limit (WEL) for flour is adhered to strictly
e) Symptoms have no correlation with length of exposure time

QUESTION 13: CARCINOGENS

Tetrachloroethylene is used in which industry?

a) Dry cleaning
b) Paper manufacture
c) Welding
d) Rubber manufacture
e) Construction

QUESTION 14: OCCUPATIONAL DISEASES

Which of the following occupational hazards is paired with the disease that it causes?

a) Crocidolite: mesothelioma
b) Oil: strimmer dermatitis
c) PVC: biliary cirrhosis
d) Mercury: epilepsy
e) Silica: extrinsic allergic alveolitis

QUESTION 15: OCCUPATIONAL DISEASES

Which of the following occupational diseases is paired with its at-risk occupation?

a) Chronic obstructive pulmonary disease (COPD): quarrying
b) Interstitial pneumonitis: baking
c) Skin cancer: metal workers
d) Penile cancer: chimney sweeper
e) Nasopharyngeal adenoma: wood workers

QUESTION 16: OCCUPATIONAL HEALTH

Which is the most common occupational health disease in the UK?

a) Depression
b) Back pain
c) Repetitive strain injury
d) Asthma
e) None of the above

QUESTION 17: OCCUPATIONAL CANCERS

Shift work is thought to be associated with which pathology?

a) Breast cancer
b) Renal carcinoma
c) Leukaemia
d) Testicular cancer
e) None of the above

QUESTION 18: SKIN DISEASES

In your occupational health clinic you see a 32-year-old gentleman who presents with lichenification on his hands after starting to work with a particular substance. You diagnose him with allergic contact dermatitis. Which of the following is incorrect with regard to allergic contact dermatitis?

a) The effects can be permanent
b) It can be diagnosed using a prick test
c) It is a type IV hypersensitivity reaction
d) Symptoms are only seen at the point of contact
e) Atopics have a lower threshold for obtaining the disease

QUESTION 19: STRESS

Which of the following is not part of the HSE guidance on work-related stress, which suggests areas where the reduction of stress is under managerial control?

a) Job suitability
b) Relationships at work
c) Rate of pay
d) Job demands
e) Organizational factors

QUESTION 20: TINNITUS

A worker is complaining of ringing in his ears. Which of the following is correct?

a) Tinnitus is almost always pathological
b) Unilateral tinnitus is likely to be noise related
c) Tinnitus can result in disturbed sleep
d) Tinnitus is not normally associated with noise exposure
e) Tinnitus is rarely disabling

QUESTION 21: HEARING

Which of the following statements is true of hearing loss?

a) Poor hearing is associated with motorcycle use
b) Hearing impairment and disability are the same
c) Noise conservation programmes are best evaluated by self-recorded audiometry
d) Hearing loss is synergistic
e) Hearing aids restore hearing to normal

QUESTION 22: HEARING

You discover that an employee has suffered from noise-induced hearing loss. Which of the following statements is true?

a) Employers have no legal duty to move employees against their wishes
b) An audiogram can be diagnostic
c) Tinnitus and hearing loss are not synergistic
d) Noise-induced hearing loss is not RIDDOR (Reporting of Injuries, Diseases and Dangerous Occurrences Regulations) reportable
e) Surveillance of other workers is not needed

QUESTION 23: RESPIRATORY SENSITIZERS

Which of the following occupations is unlikely to be exposed
to respiratory sensitizers?

a) Laboratory worker
b) Baker
c) Paint sprayer
d) Farmer
e) None of the above

QUESTION 24: RESPIRATORY SENSITIZERS

Which of the following is not a respiratory sensitizer?

a) Resin
b) Latex
c) Isocyanates
d) Sheep
e) None of the above

QUESTION 25: EPILEPSY

An employee who drives to work wants to come off his anti-epileptic
medication (he does not drive at work). He has not had a seizure for
7 years. How long should he be advised to wait before he can drive to
work after stopping his medication?

a) 3 months
b) 6 months
c) 8 months
d) 12 months
e) 14 months

QUESTION 26: SILICA

You are undertaking health surveillance on miners who are exposed to silica. Which of the following is correct?

a) Smoking and silica exposure are synergistic
b) Routine testing for TB is indicated
c) A CT chest is never indicated
d) A reduction in the percentage predicted FEV1 (forced expiratory volume in 1 second) to less than 80% of the predicted value is unlikely to be significant
e) Two sets of spirometry should be recorded as a minimum

QUESTION 27: HAVS

Which of the following statements is not true about HAVS?

a) HAVS can cause joint pain
b) A diagnosis of HAVS increases the risk of carpal tunnel syndrome
c) HAVS is generally symmetrical
d) HAVS is graded by the Stockholm criteria
e) None of the above

QUESTION 28: SKIN PROBLEMS

A 20-year-old hairdresser comes to see you with flaking and scaling of her hands made worse at work. It does not occur outside of work. Which of the following statements is correct?

a) Prick testing is indicated
b) Using gloves all day is useful in reducing her skin problems
c) Patch testing is not indicated
d) A wet work policy would not be useful
e) You should prescribe her steroids

QUESTION 29: OCCUPATIONAL ASTHMA

Mr Pryor is a baker who has just been diagnosed with occupational asthma. Management want advice on how his disease will be managed. Which is the most appropriate management plan by occupational health for the management of this patient?

a) Salbutamol when he is symptomatic
b) Respiratory protective equipment for the employee
c) Health surveillance for the other employees
d) Redeployment
e) None of the above

QUESTION 30: OCCUPATIONAL ASTHMA

A mechanic gets wheezy every time he uses two-part paint. You diagnose occupational asthma after various investigations have been undertaken. Which of the following is correct?

a) IgE is always raised in occupational asthma
b) You can get rhinitis with the condition
c) Can be diagnosed with twice daily peak flow readings for 2 weeks at home and at work
d) Does not require health surveillance of other workers
e) Is not an IIDB disease

QUESTION 31: OCCUPATIONAL ASTHMA

Which of the following occupations is not at higher risk of occupational asthma?

a) Stainless steel maker
b) Baker
c) Hairdresser
d) Shoe maker
e) None of the above

QUESTION 32: DERMATOLOGY

You see a student nurse who presents with wheals every time she puts on latex gloves. She has no systemic symptoms. This condition…

a) Is diagnosed with a patch test
b) Is a type IV sensitivity reaction
c) Is associated with anaphylaxis
d) Is commoner in patients with atopy
e) Takes weeks to evolve

QUESTION 33: PEAK FLOW

The following are the most important factors that must be taken into account when assessing peak flow:

a) Gender, age, height
b) Gender, height, weight
c) Smoking status, age, gender
d) Smoking status, recent infection, gender
e) Smoking status, age, height

QUESTION 34: UPPER LIMB DISORDERS

Which of the following is not an aid to help reduce ULDs?

a) MAC tool
b) ART tool
c) Penguin mouse
d) Joystick mouse
e) None of the above

QUESTION 35: OCCUPATIONAL DISEASE

Which agent is correctly paired with the disease it causes?

a) Cotton: hepatitis
b) Cadmium: hepatic carcinoma
c) Lead: foot drop
d) Egg: asthma
e) All of the above

QUESTION 36: OCCUPATIONAL DISEASE

Which employment is not correctly paired with the disease associated with it?

a) Cotton workers: byssanosis
b) Felt workers: psychosis
c) Carpenters: penile carcinoma
d) Tree surgeons: HAVS
e) Laboratory workers: asthma

QUESTION 37: CARCINOGENS

Benz(a)pyrene is associated with which pathology?

a) Nasal carcinoma
b) Small cell lung cancer
c) Bladder cancer
d) Scrotal carcinoma
e) Laryngeal carcinoma

ANSWERS to Effects of work on health questions

QUESTION 1: ASBESTOS EXPOSURE

You see a 60-year-old carpenter who has worked with asbestos in the past. He has had an X-ray that has been reported as showing pleural plaques. Which of the following is incorrect?

The answer is: e) Pleural plaques affect the visceral pleura

- Pleural plaques are benign, affect the parietal pleura and are common.
- Whilst they are pathognomic for asbestos exposure they are not for mesothelioma.

QUESTION 2: BLOOD-BORNE VIRUS

A student nurse comes to an NHS clinic after a needle-stick injury. She has not been vaccinated against hepatitis B. She is very worried about her risk of contracting a blood-borne virus. Her approximate risk is…

The answer is: a) 1 in 3

- The main blood-borne viruses are hepatitis B and C, and HIV.
- The risk of contracting hepatitis B is the greatest, with the risk being 1 in 3.
- The risk of contracting hepatitis C is approximately 1 in 30.
- The risk of contracting HIV is approximately 1 in 300.

QUESTION 3: DERMATITIS

Ms Pryor is setting up a hairdressing business. She wants advice on how to control the risk of dermatitis. Which of the following measures are useful for her?

The answer is: e) All of the above

Advice on the control of dermatitis can be found in the HS24 guide. This includes:
- Using barrier cream.
- Not using gloves for more than 20 minutes at a time.
- Visual and questionnaire surveillance.
- A wet work policy should outline all of the above.

QUESTION 4: DIABETES

Diabetic lorry drivers…

The answer is: d) On metformin must monitor their blood glucose at least twice a day

- Diabetic Group 2 licence holders must tell the DVLA if they take any type of medication for their illness.
- Insulin-dependent diabetics must undergo an independent medical assessment every year. They must also check their blood glucose at least two hours before getting behind the wheel and every two hours whilst driving.
- Debarring criteria include:
  - Hypoglycaemia requiring the assistance of another person occurring within the preceding 12 months.
  - No awareness of hypoglycaemic episodes.

QUESTION 5: EPILEPSY

Mr Smith has well-controlled epilepsy. He has not had a seizure in 12 years. He has not told his employers about his condition. Which of the following statements is true?

The answer is: c) If his epilepsy interferes with his ability to do his job safely then his employers may dismiss him

- He has no legal duty to disclose information about medical illnesses as long as he thinks that it will not affect his ability to do his work safely and efficiently. However, this may invalidate any insurance that his employers may provide him at work, and will not allow any reasonable adjustments that might be employed.
- His employers can ask about disabilities to make reasonable adjustments for the interview process.
- His employers could dismiss him if his epilepsy impacts on his work, if they can prove that he did not tell them and had every opportunity to do so.

- He can hold a Group 2 licence if he has not had a seizure in 10 years and does not take anti-epileptic treatment.
- Those with a diagnosis of epilepsy are not allowed to join the Armed Forces.

QUESTION 6: EPILEPSY

You see a man diagnosed with epilepsy who wants to go back to work as an HGV driver. He has been seizure-free for a number of years. How many years must he be seizure-free before he can have a Group 2 licence?

The answer is: d) 10

HGV drivers must not be on anti-epileptic medication and must be seizure-free for ten years.

QUESTION 7: OCCUPATIONAL DISEASES

Which of the following diseases is associated with coal mining?

The answer is: a) Rheumatoid arthritis

- Coal miners are susceptible to Caplan's syndrome (rheumatoid arthritis + pneumoconiosis).
- Angiosarcoma is associated with the PVC industry; bladder cancer with the rubber-making industry; COPD with silica; renal failure with working with cadmium; and asthma with lots of industries.

QUESTION 8: HAVS

You see a 35-year-old ship builder who is having difficulty picking up small objects; you suspect he has HAVS. Which of the following is correct?

The answer is: a) Smoking worsens HAVS

- HAVS comprises numbness and tingling in the fingers, reduced sensory perception, reduced dexterity, blanching, and potentially trophic changes.
- It is caused by prolonged exposure to vibration.
- Smoking worsens peripheral circulation and therefore can exacerbate symptoms.
- Suitable clothing that can help to aid circulation is useful, but is not preventative.
- Nifedipine is a treatment for improved circulation.

QUESTION 9: HEARING

You discover that a patient in a printing factory has suffered from noise-induced hearing loss. Which of the following statements is true?

The answer is: a) Employers have no legal duty to move employees against their wishes

- If the employee is given all the information about further risks to their health then still wishes to continue in their job then there is no legal obligation to relocate them.
- Those of Afro-Caribbean descent are more susceptible to noise-induced hearing loss.
- Toluene (a printing fluid) is linked to sensorineural hearing loss.
- Best practice is that workers should be informed that anonymized data are being released and be allowed to withdraw consent if they wish.

QUESTION 10: HEARING

Whilst undertaking hearing surveillance of factory workers you come across this audiogram of an employee. Which of the following statements is correct?

The answer is: c) All doctors working in occupational health can undertake hearing surveillance

- The audiogram in the question shows presbycusis.
- As always the hierarchy of control applies.
- Hearing surveillance is a legal requirement when the noise exceeds 80 dB.

Noise-induced hearing loss shows a notch at 4 kHz and/or 6 kHz:

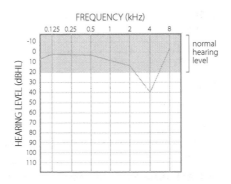

QUESTION 11: MENTAL HEALTH

You see a fireman who has been struggling at work recently. You think that he has a diagnosis of depression. Which of the following statements is correct?

The answer is: d) Night shift work may not be advisable in his case

- Presenteeism and absenteeism are associated with mental health problems.
- Occupational health physicians should not be prescribing medication, but should advise the employee to see the appropriate doctor to do so.
- The Boorman Report relates to the NHS only.
- Working at night may exacerbate mental health symptoms.
- He could work **within** the fire department in a different role, for example in management, but perhaps **not as a frontline operational fireman** due to the stressful nature of the job.

QUESTION 12: OCCUPATIONAL ASTHMA

You undertake screening in a bakery in which a case of occupational asthma has been diagnosed. You see a gentleman who has a wheeze that only occurs at work. Which of the following statements is true?

The answer is: b) Legally his employer should relocate him

- Occupational asthma is common particularly in the following occupations:
  - Bakers
  - Vets
  - Those who work with wood
  - Those who wash clothes
  - Those who spray paint.
- Respiratory protective equipment does not have any effect on the condition and the only solution is to relocate the employee.
- As his symptoms only occur at work, the implication is that his activities of daily living (ADL) are not affected and therefore he does not qualify as being disabled under the Equality Act 2010.
- Sensitizers have no WEL; employers must keep as low as is reasonably possible (ALARP).

QUESTION 13: CARCINOGENS

Tetrachloroethylene is used in which industry?

The answer is: a) Dry cleaning

Tetrachloroethylene is used in the dry cleaning industry and associated with non-Hodgkin's lymphoma, although the HSE states that the actual causal link is unknown.

QUESTION 14: OCCUPATIONAL DISEASES

Which of the following occupational hazards is paired with the disease that it causes?

The answer is: a) Crocidolite: mesothelioma

- Crocidolite is a form of asbestos.
- The other forms are: chrysotile, amosite, tremolite, anthophyllite and actinolite.

QUESTION 15: OCCUPATIONAL DISEASES

Which of the following occupational diseases is paired with its at-risk occupation?

The answer is: a) COPD: quarrying

- Quarrying is associated with exposure to sandstone.
- Sandstone contains 70–90% silica.
- Other professions at risk include the construction industry and concrete manufacture.
- Silica exposure can cause silicosis, COPD and lung cancer.

QUESTION 16: OCCUPATIONAL HEALTH

Which is the most common occupational health disease in the UK?

The answer is: b) Back pain

The HSE reports the most common cause of occupational health disease is back pain, followed by upper limb disorders and mental health problems.

QUESTION 17: OCCUPATIONAL CANCERS

Shift work is thought to be associated with which pathology?

The answer is: a) Breast cancer

According to the HSE, shift work is thought to be associated with breast cancer but more research is needed.

QUESTION 18: SKIN DISEASES

In your occupational health clinic you see a 32-year-old gentleman who presents with lichenification on his hands after starting to work with a particular substance. You diagnose him with allergic contact dermatitis. Which of the following is incorrect with regard to allergic contact dermatitis?

The answer is: b) It can be diagnosed using a prick test

- In **chromium contact dermatitis** the results are permanent.
- Allergic contact dermatitis (e.g. nickel allergy) is diagnosed by a patch test and is a **type IV hypersensitivity reaction**. It is a delayed reaction, i.e. it is chronic.
- A **patch test** is the test needed for diagnosis.
- **Atopics** are thought to have a lower threshold for allergic contact dermatitis.

There are a few differences between allergic contact dermatitis and allergic contact urticaria.

Allergic contact urticaria:
- Causes wheals.
- It can cause a systemic reaction if the allergen (e.g. latex glove) is inserted into the body.
- Is an immediate reaction, occurring within 30 minutes.
- Is a type I hypersensitivity reaction.

QUESTION 19: STRESS

Which of the following is not part of the HSE guidance on work-related stress, which suggests areas where the reduction of stress is under managerial control?

The answer is: c) Rate of pay

Work-related stress is defined as an adverse reaction to perceived lack of coping in response to pressures at work. The stress curve model suggests that there is an optimum area in which a certain level of stimulation creates the most productivity, and above this there is a continually decreasing level of productivity. Factors influencing work-related stress include high demand jobs, and lack of control and poor support at work.

The areas the HSE suggests that are under managerial control to reduce workplace stress are:
- **Job suitability** by providing job descriptions.
- **Relationships at work** by having anti-bullying and anti-harassment policies.
- **Demand at work** by change in work load.
- **Control over work** by having employee input.
- **Support at work** by encouraging things like sponsorship.
- **Organizational change** by encouraging good employer communication with employees and more employee input into organizational developments.

QUESTION 20: TINNITUS

A worker is complaining of ringing in his ears. Which of the following is correct?

The answer is: c) Tinnitus can result in disturbed sleep

- Tinnitus is common, can be the result of noise exposure, and is mainly benign.
- Warnings of other pathology include: symptoms being unilateral, and association with dizziness.
- It can result in mood and sleep disorders and can be disabling.
- Treatment is mainly with relaxation techniques, background noise and CBT.

QUESTION 21: HEARING

Which of the following statements is true of hearing loss?

The answer is: d) Hearing loss is synergistic

- HAVS is associated with motorcycle use.
- Hearing loss is associated with video gaming and gun shooting hobbies.
- Impairment is the extent of loss, and disability is the loss of function resulting from that loss.

- Noise conservation programmes are programmes evaluated by formal audiometry.
- Noise-induced hearing loss and presbyacusis are synergistic.
- Hearing aids help to increase hearing but almost always do not restore hearing to the individual's baseline.

QUESTION 22: HEARING

You discover that an employee has suffered from noise-induced hearing loss. Which of the following statements is true?

The answer is: b) An audiogram can be diagnostic

- A dip at 4 kHz and/or 6 kHz is diagnostic.
- When one worker has an occupational disease, others may also have it and therefore health surveillance is necessary.

QUESTION 23: RESPIRATORY SENSITIZERS

Which of the following occupations is unlikely to be exposed to respiratory sensitizers?

The answer is: e) None of the above

Respiratory sensitizer exposure is common in many industries. They include:
- Farmers with animals
- Lab workers and animals
- Bakers and flour
- Paint sprayers and isocyanates
- Healthcare workers and latex
- Solderers and rosin.

QUESTION 24: RESPIRATORY SENSITIZERS

Which of the following is not a respiratory sensitizer?

The answer is: a) Resin

Respiratory sensitizers:
- Animals
- Flour

- Isocyanates (found in two-part paint)
- Latex
- Rosin (found in soldering flux)
- Hardwood and softwood dust.

QUESTION 25: EPILEPSY

An employee who drives to work wants to come off his anti-epileptic medication (he does not drive at work). He has not had a seizure for 7 years. How long should he be advised to wait before he can drive to work after stopping his medication?

The answer is: b) 6 months

The DVLA medical panel recommends the licence holder should be advised not to drive from the beginning of the period of withdrawal, and for a period of six months after stopping medication. This is due to the potential risk of seizures occurring during anti-epileptic drug withdrawal.

QUESTION 26: SILICA

You are undertaking health surveillance on miners who are exposed to silica. Which of the following is correct?

The answer is: a) Smoking and silica exposure are synergistic

- Testing for TB should only be undertaken with the appropriate history and clinical symptoms, and a CT chest is reserved for those with abnormal chest X-rays.
- The HSE suggests three spirometry values taken in sequence should be recorded as a minimum.
- As silica exposure can be associated with COPD, a reduction in FEV1 and/or FVC (forced vital capacity) to below less than 80% of predicted values could be significant, and would warrant further investigation, as would successive falls in readings over the years of surveillance.

QUESTION 27: HAVS

Which of the following statements is not true about HAVS?

The answer is: c) HAVS is generally symmetrical

HAVS is a problem in industries such as the forestry industry and road working, and is due to vibration. It is also known as vibration white finger. Early signs of disease include numbness and/or pins and needles in the fingers at the end of the day; these can progress to reduced sensation, reduced dexterity, reduced grip, and blanching of the fingers.

- HAVS increases the likelihood of carpal tunnel syndrome.
- An important differential diagnosis is Raynaud's disease, which is more likely to be symmetrical.

QUESTION 28: SKIN PROBLEMS

A 20-year-old hairdresser comes to see you with flaking and scaling of her hands made worse at work. It does not occur outside of work. Which of the following statements is correct?

The answer is: c) Patch testing is not indicated

- This hairdresser has irritant dermatitis which is not immune mediated. It is caused by breaks in the skin resulting in irritation and can cause flaking and itching.
- A wet work policy is useful for people that work with water (e.g. hairdressers).
- The wet work policy outlines the use of barrier creams as well as the maximum amount of time people should be wearing gloves (max. 20 minutes at a time), as this can exacerbate the problem.
- Prick and patch testing are not indicated as this is not a hypersensitivity reaction.
- An occupational health physician should not be prescribing medication, but referring to the appropriate doctor.

QUESTION 29: OCCUPATIONAL ASTHMA

Mr Pryor is a baker who has just been diagnosed with occupational asthma. Management want advice on how his disease will be managed. Which is the most appropriate management plan by occupational health for the management of this patient?

The answer is: d) Redeployment

- Occupational asthma has a poor prognosis when the employee remains in the sensitizing environment and symptoms can be triggered by even very low amounts of the sensitizer.

- Respiratory protective equipment is useful for other employees, as well as health surveillance, and this should be undertaken promptly.
- Therefore redeployment is the best option.

QUESTION 30: OCCUPATIONAL ASTHMA

A mechanic gets wheezy every time he uses two-part paint. You diagnose occupational asthma after various investigations have been undertaken. Which of the following is correct?

The answer is: b) You can get rhinitis with the condition

- IgE response is seen when the sensitizer is a protein and would not be seen with HDI (hexamethylene diisocyanate) paint, for example.
- Those with occupational asthma can also get rhinitis, which those with non-occupational asthma do not get.
- Diagnosis requires four readings a day for at least 3 weeks to be conclusive: this is recommended by the Royal College of Physicians.
- When one worker has an occupational disease it is likely that others are already affected or will be at risk and need to be screened.
- Compensation can be granted.

QUESTION 31: OCCUPATIONAL ASTHMA

Which of the following occupations is not at higher risk of occupational asthma?

The answer is: d) Shoe maker

Egg, flour, stainless steel fumes, isocyanates, and bleaching powder are all respiratory sensitizers.

QUESTION 32: DERMATOLOGY

You see a student nurse who presents with wheals every time she puts on latex gloves. She has no systemic symptoms. This condition...

The answer is: c) Is associated with anaphylaxis

This employee is suffering from allergic contact urticaria, a localized type I reaction common in nurses, farmers and those with long-term indwelling catheters. If latex is inserted inside the body (e.g. a cannula) in people with this reaction then it causes anaphylaxis. As with all type I reactions, it is diagnosed with a prick test.

QUESTION 33: PEAK FLOW

The following are the most important factors that must be taken into account when assessing peak flow:

The answer is: a) Gender, age, height

The following is a sample peak flow chart, showing the most important variables when assessing peak flow.

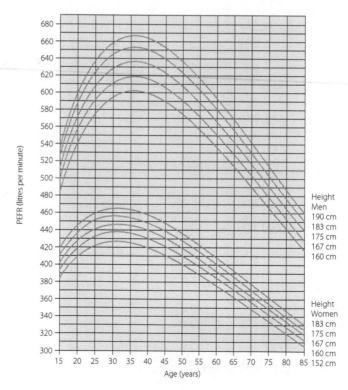

QUESTION 34: UPPER LIMB DISORDERS

Which of the following is not an aid to help reduce ULDs?

The answer is: e) None of the above

There are several tools that can be used to help those with ULD; these include a full risk assessment of the workstation and/or DSE. Tools to help with this include the Manual Handling Assessment (MAC) Tool and the Assessment of Repetitive Tasks (ART) Tool.

QUESTION 35: OCCUPATIONAL DISEASE

Which agent is correctly paired with the disease it causes?

The answer is: d) Egg: asthma

- Cadmium can cause emphysema and renal failure.
- Lead toxicity can lead to anaemia, wrist drop and constipation.
- Egg, flour and stainless steel are respiratory sensitizers and can result in asthma.

QUESTION 36: OCCUPATIONAL DISEASE

Which employment is not correctly paired with the disease associated with it?

The answer is: c) Carpenters: penile carcinoma

- Working with cotton can cause lung disease, as can working with silica and asbestos.
- Mental health problems can result from working with felt and mercury.
- Carpenters are more at risk of nasal carcinoma as part of their exposure to wood chippings.
- Forestry workers and those who use pneumatic drills are more at risk of HAVS.
- Occupational asthma can be caused by many work-related exposures including egg, flour, stainless steel and animal dander.

QUESTION 37: CARCINOGENS

Benz(a)pyrene is associated with which pathology?

The answer is: d) Scrotal carcinoma

- The classic, if now somewhat outdated example is chimney sweeps getting scrotal carcinoma.
- Benz(a)pyrene is also associated with leukaemia.

CHAPTER 3
Principles of occupational health and clinical occupational health

Which of the following is not a form of bias?

a) The Hawthorne effect
b) The healthy worker effect
c) Recall bias
d) The Bradford factor
e) Self-selection

QUESTION 2: CASE-CONTROL STUDIES

Case–control studies...

a) Are prospective studies
b) Are good for studying rare diseases
c) Are good at looking at latency of disease
d) Are good for studying prevalence
e) Cannot control for variables

QUESTION 3: RISK PHRASES

Which of the following is a risk phrase for a respiratory sensitizer?

a) G402
b) IIDB
c) R42
d) R43
e) RESP

QUESTION 4: SEQOHS

SEQOHS stands for:

a) Safe, Efficient, Quality, Occupational Health Service
b) Safe, Effective, Quality, Occupational Health Service
c) Safe, Effective, Quality, Occupational Health Standards
d) Safe, Efficient, Quality, Occupational Health Standards
e) None of the above

QUESTION 5: BRADFORD HILL CRITERIA

Which of the following is not part of the Bradford Hill criteria?

a) Strength of association
b) Temporality
c) Sensitivity
d) Specificity
e) Consistency

QUESTION 6: ERROR

What is the definition of a type 1 error?

a) True positive
b) False positive
c) True negative
d) False negative
e) None of the above

QUESTION 7: HEALTH SURVEILLANCE

Which of the following substances can you do random sampling for as part of biological health surveillance?

a) Dichloromethane
b) Carboxyhaemoglobin
c) Cadmium
d) Polychlorinated biphenyl (PCB)
e) Flour

QUESTION 8: HEALTH SURVEILLANCE

Ms Patel works with lead. Despite knowledge of the risks she refuses to undergo health surveillance. Which of the following does not apply in this case?

a) Surveillance can be done via blood tests
b) Her employment may be terminated
c) Survelllance is always needed by law
d) Acceptable lead levels are the same in all employees
e) Insisting on surveillance is an employer's duty

QUESTION 9: ERGONOMICS

Ms Sampson-Argo is undertaking an ergonomic assessment of a factory line. Which factor can an ergonomic assessment assess?

a) Time pressures
b) Adequate training
c) Adequacy of equipment
d) Support from management
e) All of the above

QUESTION 10: FITNESS FOR WORK

A lorry driver has been referred to you by management 2 months after undergoing a CABG (coronary artery bypass graft). He is asymptomatic. His GP has assessed him as being fit for work and management are being cautious. Which of the following statements is correct?

a) He can drive a lorry at present
b) Management can show preference for your medical opinion
c) He should be referred to Fit For Work
d) Your duty is to control sickness absence
e) He should be referred to the Access to Work scheme

QUESTION 11: FITNESS FOR DISCIPLINARY

Mr Johnson is due to undergo a disciplinary hearing for charges of incapability. He suddenly goes off sick with a GP note suggesting he is no longer fit to perform his working duties. You are called in to assess his capability to attend the disciplinary hearing. Which of the following is incorrect?

a) You need to assess his capability of understanding the charges
b) You need to assess his capability of answering the charges
c) The disciplinary hearing cannot be held without the employee or their representative
d) The employee does not have to attend the disciplinary in person
e) All of the above

QUESTION 12: ABSENCE MANAGEMENT

You consult with a porter with increasing sporadic absences. Which of the following statements is true?

a) Absences are generally higher in men
b) The number of absences is generally higher in the private sector
c) Doctors have the highest rates of absence in the NHS
d) The total number of working days lost is higher in older people
e) Nurses have the highest rates of absence in the NHS

QUESTION 13: DISMISSAL

Which of the following reasons is not justified as grounds for a fair dismissal?

a) Conduct
b) Capability
c) Capacity
d) Redundancy
e) All of the above

QUESTION 14: FITNESS FOR WORK

Ms Ana is a receptionist at a law firm. She recently had a myocardial infarction. She would like to come back to work and management would like an opinion on her fitness to work. What is the current guidance on when she can return to work?

a) 4–6 weeks
b) 6–8 weeks
c) 8–10 weeks
d) Once occupational health feel that she is fit to work
e) After her cardiologist feels she is fit to work

QUESTION 15: REPORTS

You receive a message that the patient you consulted with last week is not happy for the report to be sent to the employer. In this report you state that he has relapsing and remitting multiple sclerosis diagnosed in 2002, and in your medical opinion he is not currently fit for work. He states that he was diagnosed in 2000, and is adamant that he is fit for work. He does not want the report to be released unless this information is changed. Which of the following statements is the most helpful/accurate?

a) An addendum should be added to state the differences in opinion
b) An addendum should be added to state the amended date of diagnosis
c) The report cannot be changed
d) The report can be sent without those pieces of information
e) The employer cannot act without medical evidence

QUESTION 16: DRUGS AND ALCOHOL POLICY

You have been asked to provide advice on implementing a drugs and alcohol policy at work. Which of the following statements is correct?

a) Managers should be trained in any identification of misuse and treatment options
b) Consulting with employees during the instruction of a policy is a legal requirement
c) Consulting with trade unions' representatives during the instruction of a policy is a legal requirement
d) Employers can take disciplinary action against employees who do not consent to testing
e) All of the above

QUESTION 17: ABSENCE MANAGEMENT

Which of the following can help those returning to work after ill health?

a) Decreased intensity of work
b) Increased managerial support
c) Mentoring
d) Redeployment
e) All of the above

QUESTION 18: HEALTH SURVEILLANCE

Which of the following statements regarding health surveillance is incorrect?

a) It can be conducted by a questionnaire
b) It is useful for measuring exposure to isocyanates
c) It can be used to check the usefulness of the control
d) It can be a statutory requirement
e) Zinc exposure can be monitored via the urine and blood

QUESTION 19: HEALTH SURVEILLANCE

In which of the following jobs is health surveillance not mandatory?

a) Pilots
b) Divers
c) Interventional radiologists
d) Paramedics
e) None of the above

QUESTION 20: ILL HEALTH RETIREMENT

Which of the following is relevant when assessing suitability for ill health retirement?

a) Age
b) Length of service
c) Is this a terminal illness?
d) Duration
e) All of the above

QUESTION 21: OCCUPATIONAL HYGIENE

When evaluating and controlling risk, which of the following statements is correct?

a) Decreasing staff numbers can be a form of control
b) HACCP can be used
c) Hazard depends on the number of people affected and how severely
d) Blood tests are a form of direct reading
e) Increasing shift lengths is a good form of control

QUESTION 22: HEALTH SURVEILLANCE

Which of the following statements is incorrect?

a) Exposure to styrene can be monitored via its metabolite, mandelic acid
b) Exposure to lead can be monitored via its metabolite ALA (5-aminolevulinic acid)
c) Health surveillance should be undertaken by a clinician
d) Benzene can be monitored by its metabolite TTMA (trans,trans-muconic acid)
e) Health surveillance can be used to confirm adequate controls

QUESTION 23: HEALTH SURVEILLANCE

Health surveillance is an organizational requirement when working with which of the following?

a) Lead
b) Asbestos
c) Compressed air
d) Noise
e) All of the above

QUESTION 24: OCCUPATIONAL TOXICOLOGY

Which of the following statements is incorrect?

a) The time-weighted 8-hour exposure level is a measure of cumulative dose
b) The 15-minute time-weighted average is a measurement of concentration
c) Uncertainty factors take into account the unknown effects of a chemical
d) Workplace exposure limits for respiratory sensitizers can be found in the EH40
e) A high uncertainty factor value means that the unknown effect is likely to be a serious effect

QUESTION 25: TOXICOLOGY

Looking at the Dose–Response Curves, which of the following is correct?

a) B is more potent than A
b) V is the LD50
c) Y is the lowest observed level
d) Z is the threshold level
e) W is the no observable effect level

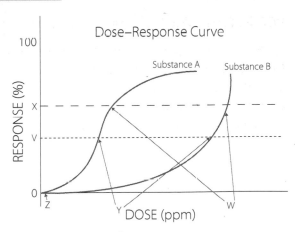

Note: ppm = parts per million

QUESTION 26: MONITORING

You are looking at general trends in concentration of substance X in individuals undergoing biological monitoring. Which of the following can affect the concentration of substance X in an individual?

a) Hand washing habits
b) Metabolism
c) Physical size
d) Hobbies
e) All of the above

QUESTION 27: MONITORING

Regarding health surveillance, which of the following statements is correct?

a) Consent is needed to undertake biological effect monitoring
b) A chest X-ray is an example of biological effect monitoring
c) Lung function tests are an example of biological effect monitoring
d) It does not always involve measuring the concentration of the hazard
e) All of the above

QUESTION 28: STATISTICS

If a study quotes a 95% confidence interval, which of the following statements is true?

a) There is a 95% chance of the true value lying outside these limits
b) There is a 5% chance of the true value lying outside these limits
c) There is a 2.5% chance of the true value lying outside these limits
d) There is a minus 5% chance of the true value lying outside these limits
e) None of the above

QUESTION 29: STATISTICS

You are asked to review a paper from the journal *Occupational Medicine*. Which of the following, with regard to statistical measurement, is incorrect?

a) The sampling error measures variability from the standard deviation
b) The case–control studies look retrospectively
c) Cohort studies measure attributable risk
d) Ecological studies do not control for confounders
e) The mode is the most represented value in a series of numbers

QUESTION 30: HEALTH SURVEILLANCE

You are asked to write a health surveillance policy for your employer. Which of the following can you, as a diploma holder in occupational health, not undertake testing of?

a) Lead
b) Flour
c) Alcohol
d) Benzodiazepine
e) None of the above

QUESTION 31: ASSESSING DISEASE

You have been asked to see a 52-year-old personal assistant with sporadic wheezy episodes whilst at work. As the next practical step you should:

a) Speak to his managers about his work environment
b) Take a detailed history
c) Inspect his workplace
d) Request his previous medical history from his general practitioner
e) Request a chest X-ray

QUESTION 32: OCCUPATIONAL TOXICOLOGY

An Occupational Toxicologist is concerned with the study of chemicals in the body. They often look at the parts of the body which the chemical hazards affect. Which of the following pairings of chemicals and affected body parts is incorrect?

a) Amosite and the lung
b) *n*-hexane and the peripheral nervous system
c) Arsenic and the skin
d) Paraquat and the liver
e) Cobalt and the kidneys

ANSWERS to Principles of occupational health and clinical occupational health questions

QUESTION 1: BIAS

Which of the following is not a form of bias?

The answer is: d) The Bradford factor

The Bradford factor is a measure of absenteeism in sickness absence management. The theory is that those who have more frequent spells of absenteeism that are shorter in nature, are more disruptive to the industry, or the productiveness of an industry, than those who have more days of absence, but fewer spells.

There are two main types of bias, **selection** bias and **information** bias.

- **Selection bias:** for example the healthy worker effect – this is when those that do an arduous manual job are likely to be healthier than those that do not. Those who are not as healthy tend to leave the organization or be put in parts of industry that are not so tough. Therefore, when studying a sub-sector of these workers, they are likely to be healthier and the results may be biased. Self-selection is also an example of this – those who choose to take part in studies may be different to the general population (e.g. they may be healthier, more likely to be exposed to a given substance, retired, or other factors) and therefore bias the results.
- **Information bias:** for example, the Hawthorne effect – this is when those studied act differently purely because they are being studied. Recall bias is also an example of this – when recalling the past, those who have had a negative effect from exposure are more likely to remember being exposed.

QUESTION 2: CASE–CONTROL STUDIES

Case–control studies…

The answer is: b) Are good for studying rare diseases

A case–control study is a retrospective study in which two groups of populations are studied – one with the disease and one without the disease. It is then looked at retrospectively, comparing those which were diseased and those which were not. Case–control studies are good for studying rare diseases, but can be subject to recall bias.

QUESTION 3: RISK PHRASES

Which of the following is a risk phrase for a respiratory sensitizer?

The answer is: c) R42

- **R43** is a skin sensitizer.
- **G402** is the document that gives guidance on health surveillance for respiratory sensitizers.
- **IIDB** is the Industrial Injuries Disablement Benefit, which gives disability money to those with prescribed diseases.
- **RESP** is a made-up phrase.

QUESTION 4: SEQOHS

SEQOHS stands for…

The answer is: b) Safe, Effective, Quality, Occupational Health Service

SEQOHS is the body that sets standards for occupational health services, giving voluntary accreditation to those whose standards are upheld. The standards involve the following:
- Business propriety
- Information governance
- Facilities
- Relationship with employers
- Relationship with workers.

The SEQOHS standards were updated in 2015 to include standards for occupational health physiotherapists, and to include the need for auditing of occupational health services and showing evidence of action taken.

QUESTION 5: BRADFORD HILL CRITERIA

Which of the following is not part of the Bradford Hill criteria?

The answer is: c) Sensitivity

The Bradford Hill criteria outline the considerations used to determine whether an agent causes a disease. The criteria are:
- Strength of association
- Temporality
- Dose–response relationship
- Analogy
- Consistency
- Coherence
- Specificity
- Experiment.

QUESTION 6: ERROR

What is the definition of a type 1 error?

The answer is: b) False positive

- Type 1 error: false positive.
- Type 2 error: false negative.

QUESTION 7: HEALTH SURVEILLANCE

Which of the following substances can you do random sampling for as part of biological health surveillance?

The answer is: c) Cadmium

Health surveillance is the monitoring at intervals of employee health, to identify early exposure to substances and therefore the early risk of disease, with the aim of being able to act before the onset of significant disease.

Health surveillance may be mandatory (e.g. in the Control of Lead at Work Regulations). It is also a way of checking that controls are adequate and also may be done if working with a substance which causes a specific disease.

In order to undertake health surveillance, you need the informed consent from the employee. The following principles must also be observed:

- There must be a chemical or substance that is known to cause a disease.
- There must be an acceptable and valid way, that is reliable and repeatable, of monitoring the exposure; for example, a liver biopsy may be a way of monitoring liver damage and the development of angiosarcoma following exposure to polyvinyl chloride, but it is not a particularly acceptable way of doing so.
- The disease must be common and if one person is affected, it must be likely that others are too.

QUESTION 8: HEALTH SURVEILLANCE

Ms Patel works with lead. Despite knowledge of the risks she refuses to undergo health surveillance. Which of the following does not apply in this case?

The answer is: d) Acceptable lead levels are the same in all employees

- Lead surveillance is a legal requirement under the Control of Lead at Work Regulations 2002.
- This can be done by a blood test or urine test
- Refusal can result in dismissal – this is a last resort
- Men and women of childbearing age have different acceptable blood lead levels as lead is teratogenic.

QUESTION 9: ERGONOMICS

Ms Sampson-Argo is undertaking an ergonomic assessment of a factory line. Which factor can an ergonomic assessment assess?

The answer is: e) All of the above

An ergonomics assessment looks at all human factors involved in the tasks at hand. These include social and psychological factors as well as physical factors.

They look at the design of tasks, the adequacy of workstations and manual handling.

QUESTION 10: FITNESS FOR WORK

A lorry driver has been referred to you by management 2 months after undergoing a CABG. He is asymptomatic. His GP has assessed him as being fit for work and management are being cautious. Which of the following statements is correct?

The answer is: b) Management can show preference for your medical opinion

- The DVLA (Driver and Vehicle Licensing Agency) guidelines state that he can drive with a Group 1 licence after 1 month and a Group 2 licence after 3 months, as long as there are no other disqualifying conditions.
- Management, not the doctor, have a duty to control sickness absence.
- Access to Work is useful for those who are likely to have a disability for 6 months or more and/or where workplace adaptations might need to be purchased.

QUESTION 11: FITNESS FOR DISCIPLINARY

Mr Johnson is due to undergo a disciplinary hearing for charges of incapability. He suddenly goes off sick with a GP note suggesting he is no longer fit to perform his working duties. You are called in to assess his capability to attend the disciplinary hearing. Which of the following is incorrect?

The answer is: c) The disciplinary hearing cannot be held without the employee or their representative

- As the occupational health physician, your role is to decide:
    - Whether the employee is capable of understanding the charges.
    - Whether the employee is capable of answering the charges – either in person or by way of a representative.
    - Whether the employee can follow procedure.
    - Whether it is ultimately in the employee's best interests for the matter to be concluded sooner, or if it should be delayed until later.
    - Whether the employee has suicidal ideation or intent.
- It needs to be taken into account that delaying the process may damage the employee's health more.
- The venue where it is held does not have to be at work – it can be a neutral venue – and the employee can be accompanied by a work colleague or union representative for support (family members or people outside of the business are not usually permitted to attend).

- In the worst case scenario where an employee cannot be contacted, if all attempts fail to reach them, then the disciplinary can be held without the employee or a representative.

QUESTION 12: ABSENCE MANAGEMENT

You consult with a porter with increasing sporadic absences. Which of the following statements is true?

The answer is: d) The total number of working days lost is higher in older people

General trends are:
- Absence is higher in women – it is thought this is because they are carers and have dependants.
- Absence is higher in the public sector compared to the private sector.
- Whilst the number of spells of absence is highest in the young, the total working days lost is higher in the elderly.
- The spells of absence are also higher in the lower grades of work.
- In the NHS, ambulance workers have the highest levels of sickness absence.
- Unemployment is associated with poor physical and mental health, and there is evidence to show that once a person has been off for over 6 months, the minority of them actually go back to work.

QUESTION 13: DISMISSAL

Which of the following reasons is not justified as grounds for a fair dismissal?

The answer is: c) Capacity

There are two types of dismissal **fair** dismissal and **unfair** dismissal.

The Approved Code of Practice outlines how a dismissal should be undertaken, including an investigation into the reasons for dismissal; writing to the employee outlining these; allowing a meeting between employee and employer with the union representative present; documenting the outcome of the meeting, and sending a copy of this to the employee; and giving the employee a chance to appeal. However, a statute suggests the following should be undertaken as a minimum:

- An investigation of the grounds for dismissal.
- The employer should have a reasonable and genuine belief that the employee is guilty.
- A dismissal of the employee is a reasonable outcome for the offence committed.

The following are the categories of **fair** dismissal:
- Conduct
- Capability
- Redundancy
- Other statutory reason.

QUESTION 14: FITNESS FOR WORK

Ms Ana is a receptionist at a law firm. She recently had a myocardial infarction. She would like to come back to work and management would like an opinion on her fitness to work. What is the current guidance on when she can return to work?

The answer is: a) 4–6 weeks

The general advice is 4–6 weeks after a myocardial infarction, 4–8 weeks after a CABG, and within a month after an angioplasty.

QUESTION 15: REPORTS

You receive a message that the patient you consulted with last week is not happy for the report to be sent to the employer. In this report you state that he has relapsing and remitting multiple sclerosis diagnosed in 2002, and in your medical opinion he is not currently fit for work. He states that he was diagnosed in 2000, and is adamant that he is fit for work. He does not want the report to be released unless this information is changed. Which of the following statements is the most helpful/accurate?

The answer is: a) An addendum should be added to state the differences in opinion

It is good practice to offer the patient the chance to see the report before the employer, or at the same time as the employer. The employee can request for imprecise factual information in the report to be changed; however, a medical opinion cannot be changed when requested by the employee. Notwithstanding this, an addendum can be added to record a difference in opinion between the employee and the occupational health physician.

Occupational health reports undergo the principle of no surprises, that is the employee should be absolutely clear about what process they are engaging in and also what information will be reported about them to a third party.

QUESTION 16: DRUG AND ALCOHOL POLICY

You have been asked to provide advice on implementing a drugs and alcohol policy at work. Which of the following statements is correct?

The answer is: e) All of the above

- When designing and implementing a drugs and alcohol policy the following should be considered:
  - Should it cover all employees?
  - Should it be a zero tolerance policy?
  - Does it respect human rights?
  - Is it fair?
  - Should testing be included?
  - Who should be testing?
  - What should be done about positive results?
  - What support is available to employees that admit to addiction or have positive results?
  - How should testing be conducted?
- Consulting with employees and their trade unions is a legal requirement under the Health and Safety (Consultation with Employees) Regulation 1996.
- Employees may raise objections to invasion of their privacy and over-zealous testing; this may be avoided by reassuring employees that managers would be trained in early identification of drugs and alcohol misuse and treatment options to avoid unfair or over-zealous testing.
- If an employer intends to take disciplinary action against those who do not consent for testing this must be clearly stated in the policy, and it is generally advisable to incorporate the need for compliance with drugs and alcohol testing within the employee contract.

QUESTON 17: ABSENCE MANAGEMENT

Which of the following can help those returning to work after ill health?

The answer is: e) All of the above

Reducing variances for those who return to work include a phased return to work, that is:
- Altering working hours.
- Limiting the activity which the person does.
- Modifying the equipment.
- Assigning them to a different workplace.
- Redeployment.
- Increasing managerial support.

QUESTION 18: HEALTH SURVEILLANCE

Which of the following statements regarding health surveillance is incorrect?

The answer is: b) It is useful for measuring exposure to isocyanates

Health surveillance is the monitoring of employee health to make sure work is not making an employee unwell, and to move a worker at signs of illness to prevent harm.
- This can be a statutory requirement and can be done via medical and non-medical methods.
- Biological monitoring can be direct or via metabolites.

QUESTION 19: HEALTH SURVEILLANCE

In which of the following jobs is health surveillance not mandatory?

The answer is: d) Paramedics

Health surveillance is mandatory under seven regulations:
- Control of Lead at Work Regulations 2002.
- Control of Noise at Work Regulations 2005.
- Control of Vibration at Work Regulations 2001.
- Work with Compressed Air Regulations 1996.
- Control of Asbestos Regulations 2012.
- Ionizing Radiation Regulations 1999.
- Substances outlined in the Control of Substances Hazardous to Health (COSHH) 2001.

QUESTION 20: ILL HEALTH RETIREMENT

Which of the following is relevant when assessing suitability for ill health retirement?

The answer is: e) All of the above

- To be considered for ill health retirement workers must be a member of a pension scheme.
- With age it can be harder to cope with illness and function normally, particularly if there are comorbidities present.
- All pension schemes have certain criteria to be fulfilled before ill health retirement can be considered, including length of service.
- Relevant treatments should have been given enough time to work.

QUESTION 21: OCCUPATIONAL HYGIENE

When evaluating and controlling risk, which of the following statements is correct?

The answer is: b) HACCP can be used

- Occupational hygiene is the study and prevention/minimization of risk at work.
- A hazard is something that has the potential to cause harm.
- The risk of harm depends on who is affected and how.
- HACCP (hazard analysis and critical control points) is a system for food hygiene with the aim of identifying hazards and placing controls to minimize risk.

QUESTION 22: HEALTH SURVEILLANCE

Which of the following statements is incorrect?

The answer is: c) Health surveillance should be undertaken by a clinician

Health surveillance does not necessarily have to be undertaken by a clinician.

There are several types of health surveillance, including:
- **Questionnaires** – these can be undertaken by the employer, with a protocol in place if a questionnaire flags up that somebody is at risk of disease due to an exposure at work.
- **Biological effect monitoring**.
- **Biological monitoring**.

Examples of biological effect monitoring include:
- Styrene via its metabolite mandelic acid.
- Lead via the enzyme ALA in the urine.

QUESTION 23: HEALTH SURVEILLANCE

Health surveillance is an organizational requirement when working with which of the following?

The answer is: e) All of the above

Health surveillance is a legal requirement when working with:
- Substances outlined in COSHH
- Lead
- Asbestos
- Compressed air
- Ionizing radiation.

QUESTION 24: OCCUPATIONAL TOXICOLOGY

Which of the following statements is incorrect?

The answer is: d) Workplace exposure limits for respiratory sensitizers can be found in the EH40

Respiratory sensitizers and carcinogens do not have a workplace exposure limit; therefore, they should be kept as low as reasonably practicable.

There are two exposure limits for different chemicals:
1. The 8-hour time-weighted average, which is a measure of cumulative dose.
2. The 15-minute time-weighted average, which is a measure of the concentration.

Occupational toxicologists study:
- The effect of chemicals on the body.
- How the chemical enters the body.

QUESTION 25: TOXICOLOGY

Looking at the Dose–Response Curves, which of the following is correct?

The answer is: c) Y is the lowest observed level

V = threshold below which individual does not respond

W = mean toxic dose (MTD) or medial lethal dose, i.e. dose at which 50% of those exposed die

X = 50% response

Y = lowest observed effect level (LOEL), i.e. lowest dose at which effects occur

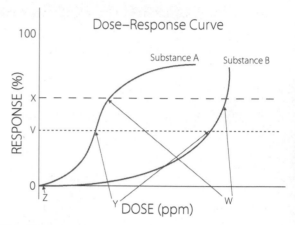

Z = no observed effect level (NOEL), i.e. at this level there are no observable effects

QUESTION 26: MONITORING

You are looking at general trends in concentration of substance X in individuals undergoing biological monitoring. Which of the following can affect the concentration of substance X in an individual?

The answer is: e) All of the above

Health surveillance can involve biological effect monitoring and biological monitoring as well as questionnaires and visual inspection.

There can be variations in exposure to the substance, and the concentration of the substance, or the effect of the substance due to:
- Physical differences, resulting in different exposures between individuals.
- Pharmacological differences between individuals (e.g. enzyme induction) resulting in different levels of metabolism within individuals.
- Different habits of an individual, for example, hobbies and whether or not they wash their hands before they eat.

QUESTION 27: MONITORING

Regarding health surveillance, which of the following statements is correct?

The answer is: e) All of the above

Biological monitoring aims to determine that an individual has been exposed to the hazard. Biological monitoring is undertaken by testing biological samples for the actual hazard or its metabolite (e.g. blood tests).

Biological effect monitoring measures the effect of the hazard on the individual who has been exposed (e.g. peak flow or lung function tests).

Examples of biological monitoring include:
- Styrene via its metabolite mandelic acid.
- Lead via the enzyme ALA in the urine.
- Lead via zinc protoporphyrin in the blood.

The time of day at which the measurement is made can be important, and can depend on when the peak time of exposure is, as well as the half-life of the substance being measured.

QUESTION 28: STATISTICS

If a study quotes a 95% confidence interval, which of the following statements is true?

The answer is: b) There is a 5% chance of the true value lying outside these limits

The 95% confidence interval (CI) indicates that the true value has a 95% chance of lying within this range. It is represented on a Forest plot as a horizontal line; a longer line means a wider CI.

QUESTION 29: STATISTICS

You are asked to review a paper from the journal *Occupational Medicine*. Which of the following, with regard to statistical measurement, is incorrect?

The answer is: c) Cohort studies measure attributable risk

The attributable risk is the number of cases with a disease attributed to an exposure – that is the difference in the rate of occurrence of a condition between an exposed population and an unexposed population.

The median number in a group of data is the middle value, the mode is the most frequent value, and the mean is the average value. The mode and the median help clarify the distribution of the data around the average value.

A case–control study is a retrospective study in which two groups of populations are studied, one with the disease and one without the disease. Then those which were exposed and those which were not, are looked at retrospectively. Case–control studies are good for studying rare diseases, but can be subject to recall bias.

Cohort studies take two groups of people and can be retrospective or prospective. Retrospectively, they are mainly looking at lessons to be learnt. Prospectively, cases are followed up to see who contracts the disease. These are particularly good at looking at the latency of disease. The measurement used in cohort studies is the relative risk.

QUESTION 30: HEALTH SURVEILLANCE

You are asked to write a health surveillance policy for your employer. Which of the following can you, as a diploma holder in occupational health, not undertake testing of?

The answer is: a) Lead

HSE appointed doctors specifically have to undertake screening for substances such as lead and asbestos. You also have to have specific training to test for occupational noise induced hearing loss. The Faculty of Occupational Medicine's guidance on alcohol and drugs states that occupational health physicians can test for alcohol and drugs, but their role has to be clearly defined and set apart from their normal occupational health physician role.

When writing a health surveillance policy the following must be covered:
- Has an appropriate risk assessment already be done?
- Who is to be screened?
- What is the justification?
- How are they going to be screened?
- How often are they going to be screened?
- Who is going to screen them?

- Informed consent must be taken from all to be screened.
- How will positive tests be actioned?
- Who will pay and be responsible for referrals?
- How will data be stored under the Data Protection Act?
- How will the results be communicated?
- How will they be done confidentially?
- How will general trends be fed back?
- How and when will health surveillance be audited?
- How will the individuals with positive results be employed?
- Who is responsible for the overall health surveillance from the health point of view and from the employer's point of view?
- What legal requirements are there for the health surveillance?
- Is there any guidance that we could follow (e.g. the MS24, which is the guidance on skin surveillance, and the G402, which is the new guidance on respiratory surveillance)?

Health surveillance should not be undertaken without a robust health surveillance policy.

QUESTION 31: ASSESSING DISEASE

You have been asked to see a 52-year-old personal assistant with sporadic wheezy episodes whilst at work. As the next practical step you should:

The answer is: b) Take a detailed history

In this scenario, taking a detailed history should come before a workplace inspection. You cannot request further information without his expressed consent and this may not be appropriate at this stage. Requesting investigations would not be your role – this would be down to his treating physician, i.e. the GP or a specialist, if you need a specialist opinion.

QUESTION 32: OCCUPATIONAL TOXICOLOGY

An Occupational Toxicologist is concerned with the study of chemicals in the body. They often look at the parts of the body which the chemical hazards affect. Which of the following pairings of chemicals and affected body parts is incorrect?

The answer is: d) Paraquat and the liver

- **Paraquat** is found in weedkillers and accumulates in the lung, causing respiratory failure.
- **Amosite** is one of the straight-fibred forms of asbestos, which accumulates in the lungs, causing asbestosis and mesothelioma, among others.
- ***n*-hexane** is found in glue solvents.
- **Cobalt** is a heavy metal which accumulates in the kidneys, causing renal failure.
- **Arsenic** causes skin cancer.

CHAPTER 4
Miscellaneous

You have been asked to provide advice on implementing a drugs and alcohol policy at work. Which of the following statements is correct?

a) A breathalyser is the most appropriate method of measuring intoxication
b) Using the chain of command ensures the integrity of the sample
c) Two samples should always be taken
d) Management should be informed of the result levels
e) All of the above

QUESTION 2: FOOD SAFETY AND HYGIENE

Which of the following statements is correct?

a) Food safety enforcement is enforced by the Health and Safety Executive (HSE)
b) The Food Safety Act covers hazard analysis and critical control points (HACCP)
c) The engineer of a food manufacturing line could be classed as a food handler
d) Food handlers must be excluded from work for 98 hours after diarrhoea and vomiting
e) All of the above

QUESTION 3: FOOD HANDLERS

For which of the following infections is microbiological clearance needed before a food handler can go back to work?

a) *Vibrio cholerae*
b) *Shigella* dysentery
c) *Salmonella* Paratyphi
d) *Salmonella* Typhi
e) All of the above

QUESTION 4: HIERARCHY OF CONTROL

You are on a site visit to a busy, noisy engineering company. You notice several methods of hazard reduction. Out of the following, which is likely to be the most effective measure of hazard reduction?

a) Purchasing new equipment
b) Enclosing workers in sound boxes
c) Increasing the distance from noisy machinery
d) Limiting the time that employees spend working near noisy machinery
e) Ear muffs

QUESTION 5: INDUSTRIAL INJURIES DISABLEMENT BENEFIT (IIDB)

Which of the following is not a compensational injury and therefore sufferers are not entitled to IIDB?

a) COPD (chronic obstructive pulmonary disease)
b) Diffuse pleural thickening
c) Pleural plaques
d) Mesothelioma
e) Asthma

QUESTION 6: HEALTHCARE WORKERS

You see a nurse who has an allergy to latex. Which of the following can be caused by latex?

a) Contact dermatitis
b) Allergic dermatitis
c) Anaphylaxis
d) Asthma
e) All of the above

QUESTION 7: LEAD

Which of the following statements is incorrect?

a) Exposure to lead can be monitored via zinc protoporphyrin levels
b) Exposure to lead can be monitored via ALA (5-aminolevulinic acid)
c) The Control of Lead at Work Regulations 2002 have different exposure levels for men and women of childbearing age
d) Constipation occurs at 60 mg/dl lead concentration
e) Irreversible effects occur at 70 mg/dl

QUESTION 8: LEAD

Ms Nightingale works with lead. Her health surveillance blood tests are normal. Which of these adverse health effects are not associated with lead exposure?

a) Constipation
b) Wrist drop
c) Teratogenicity
d) Spasticity
e) Anaemia

QUESTION 9: LIGHTING

You are asked to see several patients in a row. They all work on the same shop floor, and are complaining of headaches and eye irritation. You suspect this is due to the lighting on the shop floor. Which of the following statements is true?

a) The Management of Health and Safety at Work Regulations 1999 indicate the minimum level of lighting required
b) Incorrect lighting does not cause neck problems
c) Sick building syndrome only occurs in new buildings
d) The minimum illumination required in a room depends on what work is being done
e) An inclusion zone can be important to protect from glare

QUESTION 10: NOISE

You see a 24-year-old man who works with pneumatic drills. He has reduced hearing due to a previous hobby, and tinnitus. Which of the following is correct?

a) Tinnitus increases with age
b) Tinnitus can be exacerbated by noise
c) Hearing conservation programmes may help prevent deafness
d) Normal hearing is not needed for the majority of jobs
e) All of the above

QUESTION 11: NOISE

You assess a lady who works with loud machinery. She has had a previous tympanoplasty. She claims to be suffering from new hearing loss that she is attributing to work-related activity. Which of the following is incorrect?

a) Pre-employment audiometry should be undertaken in employees with a history of previous ear surgery
b) A history of video gaming may be relevant
c) She should not be allowed to work in a noisy environment
d) Long-term furosemide use may be relevant
e) All of the above

QUESTION 12: RADIATION

Which of the following statements is incorrect?

a) Becquerel is a unit of decay
b) Lead stops gamma rays
c) The cells most sensitive to gamma rays and X-rays are lymphocytes
d) Acute radiation syndrome is an example of a deterministic effect
e) Chronic effects of radiation include cataracts

QUESTION 13: TEMPERATURES

What is the maximum temperature that a workplace should be?

a) 20°C
b) 25°C
c) 30°C
d) 32°C
e) None of the above

QUESTION 14: THE BLACK REPORT

The Black report suggests the use of which intervention service?

a) Fit for Work
b) Access to Work
c) Employment Medical Advisory Service
d) Employee Assistance Programme
e) NHS Occupational Health Services

QUESTION 15: THERMAL COMFORT

Which of the following is not an environmental factor that contributes to thermal comfort?

a) Air temperature
b) Radiant temperature
c) Air velocity
d) Humidity
e) Metabolic heat

QUESTION 16: THE BOORMAN REPORT

Which industry does the Boorman Report relate to?

a) Law enforcement
b) Food production
c) Healthcare
d) Education
e) Alcohol distillation

QUESTION 17: HEARING CONSERVATION

Which of the following can be found in a hearing conservation programme?

a) Noise surveys
b) Audiometric testing
c) Hearing protection
d) Employee education and training
e) All of the above

QUESTION 18: WORKING AT HEIGHT

Which statement is correct?

a) Those with epilepsy should not be working at heights
b) The Work at Heights Regulations 2005 do not apply to contractors
c) Working at heights certification is always needed to work at heights
d) Collective protection should be considered above personal protection
e) Working at heights is always a safety-critical role

QUESTION 19: SUNLIGHT

You see a gardener with a new skin condition. Which of the following statements is true?

a) A sunhat is not considered as personal protective equipment (PPE)
b) Polymorphic light eruptions are commoner in men
c) Lichen sclerosis is a frictional dermatitis
d) Skin cancer can gain IIDB
e) Strimmer dermatitis is caused by chlorophyll

QUESTION 20: OLDER WORKERS

Which of the following statements regarding older workers is true?

a) Employers should undertake specific risk assessment with older workers
b) Older workers are more likely to have accidents than younger workers
c) Employers have an increased responsibility to older workers
d) There is no upper limit of retirement age
e) None of the above

QUESTION 21: HIV

A surgical junior doctor has a needle-stick injury from a patient who is HIV positive. Which of the following statements is true?

a) She cannot work as a surgeon if she is found to be HIV positive
b) Her risk of contracting HIV is approximately 1 in 30
c) To be effective, post-exposure prophylaxis should be given within 96 hours
d) The chances of transmitting the disease are lower if the patient has AIDS convergence illness
e) HIV only affects humans

QUESTION 22: ASBESTOS EXPOSURE

You have a medical student with you in your NHS occupational health clinic. You have just seen a man diagnosed with mesothelioma and the medical student is keen to learn more about what pathologies asbestos can cause. Which of the following has a relationship with asbestos exposure?

a) Ovarian cancer
b) Laryngeal cancer
c) Lung cancer
d) Diffused pleural thickening
e) All of the above

QUESTION 23: EXPOSURE-PRONE PROCEDURES (EPP)

You are working in an occupational health department within a hospital, and a colorectal surgeon has come to see you because he has recently been diagnosed with HIV. He has started his HAART (highly active antiretroviral therapy), his viral load is decreasing, and he feels well. He wants to know whether he can go back to work. Which of the following statements is incorrect?

a) A worker who is HIV positive cannot undertake EPP
b) A worker who is hepatitis B positive cannot undertake EPP
c) A worker who is hepatitis C positive cannot undertake EPP
d) All of the above
e) None of the above

QUESTION 24: DRUGS AND ALCOHOL

You are asked for a view of the drug and alcohol policy at work. Which of the following is detected in urine?

a) Alcohol
b) Amphetamines
c) TTMA
d) ALA
e) All of the above

QUESTION 25: REPORTS

You have seen a patient who has requested to see a copy of their report before their employer. You have sent them a copy of their report in the form of a written letter. They have not replied to all of your attempts to contact them to enquire whether they have decided to consent to the report being released. How long should you wait before consent is presumed and you send the report to the employer?

a) 1 day
b) 5 days
c) 10 days
d) 21 days
e) 30 days

QUESTION 26: MEDICAL REPORTS

Which of the following is not correct?

a) The principle of no surprises applies to occupational health records
b) The employer should be told what medication the employee is taking
c) You can withhold information from the employee if it is likely to be hazardous to their health
d) Consent is needed to access specialist medical records
e) None of the above

QUESTION 27: TEMPERATURE

A warehouse packer who suffers from Raynaud's disease complains that the warehouse is too cold. What is the minimum temperature requirement in a workplace?

a) 9°C
b) 13°C
c) 15°C
d) 17°C
e) 19°C

QUESTION 28: VIBRATION

You start a new job in the forestry industry and are assessing a worker's risk from vibration. Which of the following statements applies?

a) Rubber soles can help reduce vibration risks
b) Sitting and postural factors affect vulnerability to vibration
c) Early reporting of back pain is encouraged
d) Those who stand whilst operating vibrating equipment are still at risk of the effects of vibration
e) All of the above

QUESTION 29: STATISTICS

'The percentage of positive results correctly identified by a test' is the definition of which statistical term?

a) Odds ratio
b) Positive predictive value
c) Negative predictive value
d) Sensitivity
e) Specificity

QUESTION 30: NOISE

Which of the following is correct?

a) In the hierarchy of control the best way of reducing the impact of noise is to undertake engineering controls
b) The upper exposure action value of noise pressure is 112 Pa
c) A MAC chart is useful in assessing noise
d) Noise-induced hearing loss is a RIDDOR reportable disease
e) An employee must report any defects in their ear muffs

QUESTION 31: DRIVING GUIDELINES

You see a lorry driver who has been diagnosed with absence seizure epilepsy. You inform him that he cannot drive his lorry now. You tell him that he needs to inform the DVLA (Driver and Vehicle Licensing Agency), but he refuses to accept his diagnosis. What is the next step that you should take?

a) Arrange a second opinion and advise that he does not drive in the meantime
b) Discuss your concerns with his family
c) Call the DVLA immediately
d) Call the police: it is against the law for him to drive
e) Allow him to drive and explain that it is at his own risk if he has a seizure whilst driving

QUESTION 32: DVLA

You are asked to provide advice about a bus driver who has been investigated by a neurologist and has a final diagnosis of a single isolated seizure. How long must he refrain from driving a bus?

a) 2 years
b) 4 years
c) 5 years
d) 7 years
e) 10 years

QUESTION 33: DVLA

You are asked to provide advice about a mini van driver (12-seater) who has just had a transient ischaemic attack (TIA). He is worried about driving and would like to know how long he should refrain from driving. All his investigations have been satisfactory and he has no residual disability. How long must he refrain from driving?

a) 1 month
b) 6 months
c) 12 months
d) 18 months
e) 24 months

QUESTION 34: GROUP 2 LICENCE

You are asked to complete a medical for a Group 2 licence renewal for a gentleman who is fit and well. Which form should you use?

a) D4
b) MATB1
c) CR5
d) M1
e) D1

QUESTION 35: GROUP 2 LICENCE

In a line of enquiry it becomes clear that the Group 2 licence of a 55-year-old lorry driver has not been renewed. He claims not to have known that he needed to have it renewed. How often must a Group 2 licence be renewed?

a) At this age he should not be driving a Group 2 vehicle
b) Every year after the age of 40
c) Every 5 years after the age of 40
d) Every year after the age of 45
e) Every 5 years after the age of 45

QUESTION 36: TEMPERATURE

The minimum temperature in an office should normally be at least 16°C. Which regulation is this included in?

a) The Health and Safety at Work Act 1974
b) Workplace (Health, Safety and Welfare) Regulations 1992
c) Management of Health and Safety at Work Regulations 1999
d) Health and Safety (Display Screen Equipment) Regulations 1992
e) None of the above

QUESTION 37: METALS

Which of the following agents is linked with mental health disease?

a) Mercury
b) Cadmium
c) Tungsten
d) Zinc
e) Silver

QUESTION 38: GLOVES

A 20-year-old theatre nurse comes to see you with dermatitis. What is the maximum length of time that she should be wearing gloves for continuously?

a) 20 minutes
b) 40 minutes
c) 60 minutes
d) 80 minutes
e) There is no maximum time length

QUESTION 39: MANUAL HANDLING

The MAC is a useful tool in risk assessment. Which of the following is incorrect?

a) A task classed as red indicates the highest level of risk
b) Part of the MAC assessment assesses floor conditions
c) The MAC is not designed to assess risks associated with workplace upper limb disorders
d) MAC stands for Manual Handling Assessment Chart
e) The maximum load two people should lift together should be less than 35 kg

QUESTION 40: MANUAL HANDLING

You are asked about the MAC assessment. Which of the following is incorrect?

a) Psychosocial factors are not assessed in this assessment
b) The MAC is not appropriate for some manual handling operations
c) The MAC is useful in assessing risks associated with workplace upper limb disorders
d) The MAC assesses environmental factors
e) Its use does not comprise a full risk assessment

QUESTION 41: COLD STRESS

A cold worker is noticed to be shivering at work. Which of the following is correct?

a) The HSE does not issue specific requirements on cold working
b) Confusion is a sign of hypothermia
c) Encouraging the drinking of hot drinks will not help cold workers
d) Cold stress always involves shivering
e) None of the above

QUESTION 42: FORKLIFT TRUCK DRIVERS

A potential new employee as a forklift truck driver has a history of angina. It is well controlled and he has not had any symptoms for 2 years. How long must he refrain from driving a forklift truck?

a) No restriction
b) 6 months
c) 12 months
d) 18 months
e) He cannot drive a forklift truck with his medical history

QUESTION 43: RADIATION

With regard to radiation, which of the following statements is correct?

a) All non-ionizing radiation is not harmful
b) There are no immediate effects of exposure to radiation
c) Dose-related effects are entitled 'stochastic effects'
d) Radiation obeys the same inverse square law as noise
e) Those knowingly exposed to radiation should always wear PPE

QUESTION 44: GROUP 2 LICENCE

Which of the following medical problems would not result in a Group 2 driving licence being revoked?

a) Blood pressure: 175/95
b) Multiple sclerosis
c) Lung cancer
d) Monocular vision
e) Ménière's disease

QUESTION 45: DVLA

You are asked to provide advice regarding a bus driver who has been investigated by a neurologist and has a final diagnosis of a single isolated seizure. How long must he refrain from driving his car to work?

a) 6 months
b) 1 year
c) 5 years
d) 7 years
e) 10 years

QUESTION 46: REPORTS

You have seen a patient who has requested to see a copy of their report before their employer. You have sent it to them via email. They have not replied to your emails asking whether they have decided to consent to the report being released. How long should you wait before consent is presumed?

a) 24 hours
b) 48 hours
c) 72 hours
d) 21 days
e) 30 days

ANSWERS to Miscellaneous questions

QUESTION 1: DRUGS AND ALCOHOL POLICY

You have been asked to provide advice on implementing a drugs and alcohol policy at work. Which of the following statements is correct?

The answer is: c) Two samples should always be taken

- A blood test for alcohol levels is more appropriate for quantification of results – a breathalyser could be used as a first-line investigation.
- Two samples should always be taken so that there can be one sample sent to an independent lab for testing if the result is disputed.
- Management should be informed of the result (i.e. whether it is positive or negative) and nothing else – data passed on should be kept to a minimum.
- Using a 'chain of custody' ensures the integrity of the sample.

QUESTION 2: FOOD SAFETY AND HYGIENE

Which of the following statements is correct?

The answer is: c) The engineer of a food manufacturing line could be classed as a food handler

A definition of a food handler is anyone that is involved in the manufacture of raw food. This could involve those retailing it, preparing it and transporting it.
- Food hygiene is enforced by environmental hygiene officers – **not** the HSE.
- HACCP is governed by the EC (European Commission) regulations **not** the Food Safety Act.
- Food handlers are required to be absent from work until they are 48 hours clear of diarrhoea and vomiting. They are also obligated to report illness, and follow correct food hygiene policies; they have clear reporting procedures and a no blame policy, with no financial penalty policy.

- Also covered on the EC Regulation of foodstuffs (that HACCP is governed by):
  - The need for pest control, waste control and training for staff on hygiene.
  - When and how to report illness.
  - The temperature of high risk food – if it is meant to be hot, food should be above 63°C, and if cold should be below 8°C.

QUESTION 3: FOOD HANDLERS

For which of the following infections is microbiological clearance needed before a food handler can go back to work?

The answer is: e) All of the above

Food handlers are trained when to report illness and when to stay off work, as well as the appropriate food hygiene measures to use when handling food. A food handler is anyone that directly engages in the handling of food, or who handles surfaces likely to come into contact with food, for a food business.

Workers with the following infections require microbiological clearance (i.e. three negative stool samples) before they can go back to work:
- Verotoxin-producing *Escherichia coli* (VTEC)
- *Vibrio cholerae*
- *Salmonella* Typhi
- *Salmonella* Paratyphi
- *Shigella* dysentery.

QUESTION 4: HIERARCHY OF CONTROL

You are on a site visit to a busy, noisy engineering company. You notice several methods of hazard reduction. Out of the following, which is likely to be the most effective measure of hazard reduction?

The answer is: a) Purchasing new equipment

New equipment is likely to be more noise efficient and therefore the best. This is an example of substitution in the hierarchy of control.

The most effective method of controlling a hazard is:
- **Elimination**, for example, getting rid of a process that can be termed harmful.
- Followed by **substitution**, for example, by purchasing new equipment.

- Followed by **engineering controls**, such as using sound boxes.
- Followed by **administration control**, for example, job rotation – limiting time around noisy machinery.
- At the bottom of the hierarchy control is **personal protective equipment**.

QUESTION 5: IIDB

Which of the following is not a compensational injury and therefore sufferers are not entitled to IIDB?

The answer is: c) Pleural plaques

- Asbestos exposure can cause COPD, diffuse pleural thickening, and mesothelioma – all of which can alter lung function.
- Occupational asthma can also be compensated.

QUESTION 6: HEALTHCARE WORKERS

You see a nurse who has an allergy to latex. Which of the following can be caused by latex?

The answer is: e) All of the above

Natural rubber latex proteins have the potential to cause all of the above. The amount of latex exposure needed to induce sensitization is unknown. Once sensitization has taken place, further exposure to the substance, even at low levels, may cause a reaction. The HSE suggests that gloves used should be single use and powder free to reduce the chance of sensitization.

QUESTION 7: LEAD

Which of the following statements is incorrect?

The answer is: e) Irreversible effects occur at 70 mg/dl

There is lots of legislation surrounding lead:
- Exposure to lead and health surveillance regarding lead can only be undertaken by an HSE-appointed doctor.
- The Control of Lead at Work Regulations 2002 state different exposure levels for men and women of childbearing age due to the teratogenic effects of lead.

- Above the work exposure limits, an employee must be removed from exposure.
- At 60 mg/dl, a person may experience constipation.
- At 80 mg/dl, an employee will experience irreversible effects, such as wrist drop. They can also experience anaemia and decreased consciousness at this level.

QUESTION 8: LEAD

Ms Nightingale works with lead. Her health surveillance blood tests are normal. Which of these adverse health effects is not associated with lead exposure?

The answer is: d) Spasticity

Lead can cause different effects at different exposure levels:
- Headaches
- Tiredness
- Irritability
- Constipation
- Nausea
- Stomach pains
- Anaemia
- Weight loss
- Wrist drop
- Teratogenicity.

QUESTION 9: LIGHTING

You are asked to see several patients in a row. They all work on the same shop floor, and are complaining of headaches and eye irritation. You suspect this is due to the lighting on the shop floor. Which of the following statements is true?

The answer is: d) The minimum illumination required in a room depends on what work is being done

The Management of Health and Safety at Work Act 1999 covers the need for a risk assessment. The Workplace (Health, Safety and Welfare) 1992 Regulations outline environmental and lighting minimum requirements.
- Poor lighting can cause neck injuries, eye strain, headaches, and sick building syndrome (which occurs in new and refurbished buildings – the occupants get fatigue and eye strain).

- Unhelpful lighting effects include flickering, glare and poor perception of colour.
- Problems can also occur from the incorrect installation, maintenance and disposal of lighting.

The minimum lighting requirements include:
- Level of illumination – which depends on the work being done; the speed of the work being done (or that it is required to be done at); and the age of the person undertaking it.
- Appropriate illumination ratios – which is the difference between brightness in two places.
- A glare exclusion zone.

QUESTION 10: NOISE

You see a 24-year-old man who works with pneumatic drills. He has reduced hearing due to a previous hobby, and tinnitus. Which of the following is correct?

The answer is: e) All of the above

Tinnitus increases with age and with hearing loss, and can be exacerbated by noise and the cold.

Hearing conservation programmes are put in place by employers to help preserve hearing.

QUESTION 11: NOISE

You assess a lady who works with loud machinery. She has had a previous tympanoplasty. She claims to be suffering from new hearing loss that she is attributing to work-related activity. Which of the following is incorrect?

The answer is: c) She should not be allowed to work in a noisy environment

- She is likely to be considered disabled and reasonable adjustments should be made to allow her to work in this environment.
- Hobbies such as video gaming and shooting may cause hearing loss.
- Pre-employment audiometry is needed in a number of people working in a noisy environment, including those who have had previous ear surgery and previous employment in noisy environments.
- Ototoxic drugs include gentamicin and furosemide.

QUESTION 12: RADIATION

Which of the following statements is incorrect?

The answer is: b) Lead stops gamma rays

- Gamma rays and X-rays are attenuated by lead – **not stopped** by lead.
- Alpha particles (helium nuclei) are stopped by skin and paper.
- Beta particles (electrons) are stopped by aluminium.
- A becquerel is a unit of decay; a gray (J/kg) is the unit of dose; a sievert is the unit of equivalent dose (i.e. dose × weighting effect of radiation).
- Acute radiation syndrome is deterministic – that is, it depends on the amount of radiation received, and it has a threshold effect and a dose–response curve.

The lower doses of radiation have an effect on the haematopoietic system, with higher doses having an effect on the gastrointestinal system and central nervous system.

Longer term or chronic effects include:
- Malignancy (a stochastic effect)
- Cataracts
- Sterility.

The cells most affected by ionization and radiation are the lymphocytes, with the haematopoietic progenitor cells and the gonads also being sensitive.

QUESTION 13: TEMPERATURES

What is the maximum temperature that a workplace should be?

The answer is: e) None of the above

- The Workplace (Health, Safety and Welfare) Regulations 1992 place a legal obligation on employers to provide a reasonable temperature in the workplace.
- Nevertheless, there is no maximum temperature that is stated.
- However, an individual's thermal comfort as well as heat stress should be taken into account in the workplace.

QUESTION 14: THE BLACK REPORT

The Black report suggests the use of which intervention service?

The answer is: a) Fit for Work

Working for a Healthier Tomorrow is a report by Dame Carol Black:
- It outlines the impact of sickness on the economy.
- It suggests an early intervention service to help those on sickness absence to avoid long-term sickness and get back to work as early as possible.
- The Fit for Work service is a multidisciplinary team (MDT) which is case managed, in theory providing an individual plan based on the patient's individual needs to get them back into work.

QUESTION 15: THERMAL COMFORT

Which of the following is not an environmental factor that contributes to thermal comfort?

The answer is: e) Metabolic heat

- Thermal comfort describes a person's state of comfort at a certain temperature (i.e. not uncomfortably hot or cold).
- Metabolic heat is not an environmental factor but a physical factor. The more work we do, the more heat we produce, and therefore we can overheat.
- Environmental factors include:
  - Air temperature
  - Radiant temperature
  - Air velocity
  - Humidity.

QUESTION 16: THE BOORMAN REPORT

Which industry does the Boorman Report relate to?

The answer is: c) Healthcare

- The Boorman Report is about the health and well-being of NHS staff.
- It is written by one of the diploma's examiners – Dr Steve Boorman.

The critical areas that each of the recommendations focus on are as follows:

- Organizational behaviours and performance improvement by the development of prevention-centred approaches to health and well-being and equipping leaders and managers.
- Achieving an exemplary service by improving staff engagement and by encouraging staff to be engaged in the health and well-being strategy and effective early intervention.
- Embedding health and well-being in NHS systems and infrastructure by addressing national and local issues such as the inclusion of health and well-being in the NHS.

QUESTION 17: HEARING CONSERVATION

Which of the following can be found in a hearing conservation programme?

The answer is: e) All of the above

Hearing conservation programmes are designed to minimize/prevent noise-induced hearing loss.

QUESTION 18: WORKING AT HEIGHT

Which statement is correct?

The answer is: d) Collective protection should be considered above personal protection

- The Working at Height Regulations apply to any surface where, if there was no protection in place, a person could fall and cause serious injury to themselves or others.
- The majority of workplaces at height, or with dangerous machinery, should be suitably protected and not present a problem for a person with epilepsy.
- Those who work for less than 30 minutes at height do not need to be certified to do so.

QUESTION 19: SUNLIGHT

You see a gardener with a new skin condition. Which of the following statements is true?

The answer is: d) Skin cancer can gain IIDB

- Sunlight can cause a range of pathologies including:
  - Phototoxic dermatitis (strimmer dermatitis) which is caused by sap.
  - Polymorphic light eruption.
  - Skin cancer.
- Skin cancers are commoner in those who work outside and in the forces, and in some cases gains IIDB.
- Lichen sclerosis has no relation to sunlight, and lichen planus is a frictional dermatitis.
- PPE can include clothing (as it protects from sunlight) and steel-capped shoes, as well as the more obvious earmuffs and eye masks.

QUESTION 20: OLDER WORKERS

Which of the following statements regarding older workers is true?

The answer is: d) There is no upper limit of retirement age

Older workers, pregnant workers and younger workers (under 18) are considered to be more vulnerable than other workers, and special consideration is sometimes needed when dealing with their employment.

QUESTION 21: HIV

A surgical junior doctor has a needle-stick injury from a patient who is HIV positive. Which of the following statements is true?

The answer is: e) HIV only affects humans

- The risk of contracting HIV is approximately 1 in 300.
- Risk factors which increase the likelihood of HIV transmission include:
  - Donor blood from somebody with a recent seroconversion illness.
  - Donor blood with a high viral load.
  - A deep injury.
  - The needle penetrates an artery.
- Post-exposure prophylaxis should be given within two hours ideally, but can be given up to 72 hours post-exposure.

QUESTION 22: ASBESTOS EXPOSURE

You have a medical student with you in your NHS occupational health clinic. You have just seen a man diagnosed with mesothelioma and the medical student is keen to learn more about what pathologies asbestos can cause. Which of the following has a relationship with asbestos exposure?

The answer is: e) All of the above

Asbestos exposure can cause the following diseases:
- **Pleural plaques** – which are pathognomic of asbestos exposure, but do not signify an increased risk of mesothelioma.
- **Pleural effusions.**
- **Diffuse pleural thickening** – this is a restrictive disease and patients can claim IDB4.
- **Lung cancer** – unfortunately asbestos exposure is synergistic with smoking exposure.
- **Mesothelioma.**
- **Ovarian carcinoma.**
- **Laryngeal cancer/carcinoma.**
- **Asbestosis.**

QUESTION 23: EXPOSURE-PRONE PROCEDURES

You are working in an occupational health department within a hospital, and a colorectal surgeon has come to see you because he has recently been diagnosed with HIV. He has started his HAART treatment, his viral load is decreasing, and he feels well. He wants to know whether he can go back to work. Which of the following statements is incorrect?

The answer is: d) All of the above

There have been recent changes in the Department of Health guidelines – these now state that, under certain conditions, employees who are HIV positive can undertake EPP if they fulfil certain criteria. There is also long-standing guidance on employees with hepatitis B and hepatitis C, and they can undertake EPP as long as they also fulfil certain criteria – these can be found on the Department of Health website.

QUESTION 24: DRUGS AND ALCOHOL

You are asked for a view of the drug and alcohol policy at work. Which of the following is detected in urine?

The answer is: e) All of the above

The following drugs can be detected in urine:
- Alcohol
- Cocaine
- Cannabis
- Amphetamines
- Heroin
- Morphine.

ALA is an enzyme used to detect lead in the body.

TTMA (trans,trans-muconic acid) is a metabolite of benzene used in health surveillance.

QUESTION 25: REPORTS

You have seen a patient who has requested to see a copy of their report before their employer. You have sent them a copy of their report in the form of a written letter. They have not replied to all of your attempts to contact them to enquire whether they have decided to consent to the report being released. How long should you wait before consent is presumed and you send the report to the employer?

The answer is: b) 5 days

There is no regulation governing how long one should wait before presuming consent, but agreed gold standard industry practice states that 5 days must elapse if the report has been sent by hard copy (in the post). This should not be confused with the **Access to Medical Records Act 1988** which does not apply to occupational health professionals.

QUESTION 26: MEDICAL REPORTS

Which of the following is not correct?

The answer is: b) The employer should be told what medication the employee is taking

Expressed consent is needed to gain access to specialist medical reports and GP medical reports about the employee. The Access to Medical Reports Act 1988 gives the patient the right to see medical reports prepared by a doctor responsible for their care for employment and insurance purposes.

Occupational health reports do not fall within the Access to Medical Records Act 1998, but they undergo the principle of no surprises – that is, the employee should be absolutely clear about what process they are engaging in and also what your opinion is.

Regarding the nature of your reports – information given to employers must be justifiable, necessary and to a minimum. This often means that the exact nature of the medication does not need to be disclosed – only that the patient is on the appropriate medication for their illness and is not experiencing any side effects.

QUESTION 27: TEMPERATURE

A warehouse packer who suffers from Raynaud's disease complains that the warehouse is too cold. What is the minimum temperature requirement in a workplace?

The answer is: b) 13°C

Under the Workplace (Health, Safety and Welfare) Regulations there is a legal obligation on employers to provide a 'reasonable' temperature in the workplace.

It suggests that the minimum temperature in a workplace should normally be at least 16°C. If the work involves rigorous physical effort, the temperature should be at least 13°C.

QUESTION 28: VIBRATION

You start a new job in the forestry industry and are assessing a worker's risk from vibration. Which of the following statements applies?

The answer is: e) All of the above

There are many vibrational health issues including hand arm vibration syndrome (HAVS) and whole body vibration. Controls may involve:
- Checking driving seats to ensure that they are well sprung and give adequate support.
- Fitting suspension seats to vehicles with suspended driver's cabs.

- Choosing a suitable vehicle or machine for the ground conditions and activity.
- Making sure vehicles are well maintained, including suspension systems.
- Providing information and advice on safe posture, sitting position and the use of vehicles and machinery.
- Encouraging the early reporting of back pain and discomfort.

For operators who have to stand while operating vibrating machinery, control may involve:
- Operating the machine remotely from a vibration-free area.
- Mounting fixed machinery on anti-vibration mounts.
- Using rubber mats and providing shoes with thick rubber soles.

QUESTION 29: STATISTICS

'The percentage of positive results correctly identified by a test' is the definition of which statistical term?

The answer is: d) Sensitivity

Sensitivity can also be defined as the percentage of true positives in a sample:

$$\text{sensitivity} = \text{true positives}/(\text{true positives} + \text{false positives})$$

Specificity is the number of negative results correctly identified from a sample (or the percentage of true negatives).

QUESTION 30: NOISE

Which of the following is correct?

The answer is: e) An employee must report any defects in their ear muffs

- In the hierarchy of control, elimination is the top of the hierarchy, then substitution, then engineering controls.
- The upper exposure value of noise pressure is 140 Pa.
- MAC charts are used in ergonomic assessments.
- Noise-induced hearing loss is not a RIDDOR (Reporting of Injuries, Diseases, and Dangerous Occurrences Regulations) reportable disease.
- Under PPE Regulations, defects in PPE must be reported.

QUESTION 31: DRIVING GUIDELINES

You see a lorry driver who has been diagnosed with absence seizure epilepsy. You inform him that he cannot drive his lorry now. You tell him that he needs to inform the DVLA, but he refuses to accept his diagnosis. What is the next step that you should take?

The answer is: a) Arrange a second opinion and advise that he does not drive in the meantime

The General Medical Council (GMC) has issued draft guidelines applicable to such circumstances (www.gmc.org.uk), which state:

- The driver is legally responsible for informing the DVLA about such a condition or treatment. The doctor should explain to the patient:
  - That the condition may affect their ability to drive.
  - That they have a legal duty to inform DVLA about the condition.
- If a patient refuses to accept the diagnosis, or the effect of the condition of their ability to drive, you can suggest and arrange a second opinion. You should advise the patient not to drive in the meantime.
- If a patient continues to drive when they may not be fit to do so, you should make every reasonable effort to persuade them to stop. As long as the patient agrees, you may discuss your concerns with their relatives, friends or carers.
- If you do not manage to persuade the patient to stop driving, or you discover that they are continuing to drive against your advice, you should contact the DVLA immediately.
- Before contacting the DVLA, you should try to inform the patient of your decision to disclose personal information. You should also inform the patient in writing once you have done so. Source: General Medical Council

QUESTION 32: DVLA

You are asked to provide advice about a bus driver who has been investigated by a neurologist and has a final diagnosis of a single isolated seizure. How long must he refrain from driving a bus?

The answer is: c) 5 years

DVLA guidelines state that a person with a single isolated seizure investigated by a neurologist with a yearly risk of <2% of a seizure, who is not on medication, can drive with a Group 2 licence after 5 years, provided they do not have another seizure.

QUESTION 33: DVLA

You are asked to provide advice about a mini van driver (12-seater) who has just had a TIA. He is worried about driving and would like to know how long he should refrain from driving. All his investigations have been satisfactory and he has no residual disability. How long must he refrain from driving?

The answer is: c) 12 months

Any driver driving a vehicle with over nine seats needs a Group 2 licence. The guidelines state that a Group 2 driver who has had a single TIA should have their licence revoked for 12 months. For a Group 1 licence holder they should not drive for one month.

QUESTION 34: GROUP 2 LICENCE

You are asked to complete a medical for a Group 2 licence renewal for a gentleman who is fit and well. Which form should you use?

The answer is: a) D4

- The D4 is the official DVLA form for Group 2 licence renewals.
- D1 is for Group 1 drivers reapplying for their licence after a medical condition.
- CR5 is the form for the DVLA to report mental health conditions.
- CR5 is part 2 of the cremation form.
- MATB1 is for maternity.

QUESTION 35: GROUP 2 LICENCE

In a line of enquiry it becomes clear that the Group 2 licence of a 55-year-old lorry driver has not been renewed. He claims not to have known that he needed to have it renewed. How often must a Group 2 licence be renewed?

The answer is: e) Every 5 years after the age of 45

For Group 2 vehicles the licence must be renewed every 5 years after the age of 45 until the age of 65, and from then on it must be annually.

QUESTION 36: TEMPERATURE

The minimum temperature in an office should normally be at least 16°C. Which regulation is this included in?

The answer is: b) Workplace (Health, Safety and Welfare) Regulations 1992

These regulations outline the minimum requirements needed to be undertaken by the employer to provide an adequate working environment. They include:

- A minimum temperature of 16°C (13°C in a manual work area). There is no maximum temperature limit.
- Minimum workplace size.
- Need for restrooms.
- Need for toilets.
- Need for an area for breastfeeding.
- The **Health and Safety at Work Act 1974** is an **Act** and not a Regulation.
- The **Health and Safety (Display Screen Equipment) Regulations 1992** state the minimum requirements for a workstation, including the environment, equipment (including chairs and keyboards), and the need for risk assessments of the individual and the job.
- The **Management of Health and Safety at Work Regulations 1999** outline the need for risk assessments and health surveillance amongst other things.

QUESTION 37: METALS

Which of the following agents is linked with mental health disease?

The answer is: a) Mercury

Mercury is associated with psychosis – hence the 'Mad Hatter', as it was used in hat making!

Cadmium is associated with emphysema; tungsten with giant cell pneumonia; silver with argyria; and zinc oxide fumes can cause metal fume fever.

QUESTION 38: GLOVES

A 20-year-old theatre nurse comes to see you with dermatitis. What is the maximum length of time that she should be wearing gloves for continuously?

The answer is: a) 20 minutes
- Those who wear gloves should use barrier creams.
- The maximum amount of time that people should be wearing gloves continuously is 20 minutes. Wearing them for longer periods can exacerbate dermatitis, but keeping below this limit can be difficult in practice.

QUESTION 39: MANUAL HANDLING

The MAC is a useful tool in risk assessment. Which of the following is incorrect?

The answer is: a) A task classed as red indicates the highest level of risk

The MAC assessment tool is the Manual Handling Assessment Chart used in assessing risks in manual handling.

The **Manual Handling Operations Regulations 1992** set out a clear hierarchy of measures for dealing with risk likely to cause harm from manual handling.

There are three types of assessment that can be carried out with the MAC:
- Lifting operations
- Carrying operations
- Team handling operations.

Risks can be classified into:
- GREEN – low level of risk.
- AMBER – medium level of risk.
- RED – high level of risk – prompt action needed.
- PURPLE – very high level of risk – such operations may represent a serious risk of injury.

QUESTION 40: MANUAL HANDLING

You are asked about the MAC assessment. Which of the following is incorrect?

The answer is: c) The MAC is useful in assessing risks associated with workplace upper limb disorders

The MAC assessment tool is the Manual Handling Assessment Chart used in assessing risks in manual handling.
- Psychosocial factors, including vulnerable workers should also be assessed in manual handling.

- The MAC is not appropriate for some manual handling operations, for example, those that involve pushing and pulling. It is also not used for upper limb disorders – the Assessment of Repetitive Tasks (ART) tool is used for this.
- Other factors looked at include postural constraints, grips involved, and arm position when lifting.

QUESTION 41: COLD STRESS

A cold worker is noticed to be shivering at work. Which of the following is correct?

The answer is: a) The HSE does not issue specific requirements on cold working

The HSE does not issue specific guidance on cold stress.

However, it suggests the following can help:
- Appropriate personal protective equipment.
- Provide mobile facilities for warming up, and encourage the drinking of warm fluids such as soup or hot drinks.
- More frequent rest breaks are useful.
- Educate workers about recognizing the early symptoms of cold stress.

Cold stress symptoms include:
- Early symptoms:
  - Shivering
  - Fatigue
  - Loss of coordination
  - Confusion and disorientation.
- Late symptoms:
  - No shivering
  - Blue skin
  - Dilated pupils
  - Slowed pulse and breathing
  - Loss of consciousness.

QUESTION 42: FORKLIFT TRUCK DRIVERS

A potential new employee as a forklift truck driver has a history of angina. It is well controlled and he has not had any symptoms for 2 years. How long must he refrain from driving a forklift truck?

The answer is: a) No restriction

For angina, forklift truck operation should cease until satisfactory control of symptoms is achieved. It will be a bar, however, if angina occurs during forklift truck operation, or at rest, or if medication causes undesirable side effects that interfere with forklift truck operation.

QUESTION 43: RADIATION

With regard to radiation, which of the following statements is correct?

The answer is: d) Radiation obeys the same inverse square law as noise

- Deterministic effects are characterized by being dose-related and having a threshold before an effect can be seen.
- Stochastic effects occur at random.
- Examples of damaging non-ionizing radiation include laser and infrared light, which can have a heating effect on the body.
- Doubling the distance from the radiation source halves the concentration/dose.
- Acute effects from radiation include acute radiation sickness.

QUESTION 44: GROUP 2 LICENCE

Which of the following medical problems would not result in a Group 2 driving licence being revoked?

The answer is: a) Blood pressure: 175/95

A Group 2 licence will be refused in the following cases:
- Within three months of a coronary artery bypass graft.
- Uncontrolled angina, heart failure or cardiac arrhythmia.
- Implanted cardiac defibrillator.
- Hypertension where the blood pressure is persistently ≥180 systolic and/or ≥100 diastolic.

- A stroke or TIA within the last 12 months.
- Ménière's disease, or any other sudden and disabling dizziness or vertigo within the past year, with a liability to recurrence.
- Major brain surgery and/or recent severe head injury with serious continuing after-effects or a likelihood of causing seizures.
- Parkinson's disease, multiple sclerosis or other chronic neurological disorders with symptoms likely to affect safe driving.
- Dementia.
- Lung cancer.

QUESTION 45: DVLA

You are asked to provide advice regarding a bus driver who has been investigated by a neurologist and has a final diagnosis of a single isolated seizure. How long must he refrain from driving his car to work?

The answer is: a) 6 months

As the occupational physician, issues around getting to work may be something that you need to consider.

QUESTION 46: REPORTS

You have seen a patient who has requested to see a copy of their report before their employer. You have sent it to them via email. They have not replied to your emails asking whether they have decided to consent to the report being released. How long should you wait before consent is presumed?

The answer is: b) 48 hours

There is no regulation governing how long one should wait before presuming consent, but agreed gold standard industry practice states that 48 hours must elapse if the report has been sent by email. This should not be confused with the Access to Medical Records Act 1988, which does not apply to OH professionals.

CHAPTER 5
Mock exam

You see a 20-year-old girl whose fitness to undertake a teaching degree you have been asked to assess. She has a past history of anorexia, and was admitted against her will into an eating disorders clinic 2 years ago. She tells you that she left of her own accord after 2 weeks. She tells you that since then she has completed her Duke of Edinburgh Gold Award and has been feeling well. She denies any ongoing problems. She looks to be of a normal BMI. She refuses to be weighed. She appears enthusiastic about her course.

a) You should declare her unfit for her role
b) Her GP should be contacted for further information
c) A psychiatric second opinion should be sought
d) You should declare her fit for role with adjustments
e) A WRAP (Wellbeing Recovery Action Plan) should be suggested

QUESTION 2: CHRONIC OBSTRUCTIVE PULMONARY DISEASE (COPD)

You see a 67-year-old lunchtime and playground supervisor with COPD applying for ill health retirement. She currently works 7 hours a week at a primary school. Her job involves handing out school meals and supervising the children whilst they eat, for one hour a day. She has an exercise tolerance of 20 metres "on a good day" but declares no exacerbations in the last 2 years. She is not on any oxygen but is on maximal other medical therapies, which is confirmed by the respiratory specialist's letter confirming stage 4 COPD and a FEV_1 of <30%. She tells you that she has no other skills to be able to do another job.

The criteria for ill health retirement require fulfilment of the following:

1) She has an infirmity of body or mind rendering her unable to do her contractual role;
2) She is not immediately fit for other gainful employment due to ill health for 12 consecutive months.

a) You should write to the respiratory physician for a view on whether long-term oxygen therapy (LTOT) would be appropriate to render her able to do another job
b) This lady meets the criteria for ill health retirement
c) You should declare her fit for alternative work (redeployment)
d) She can be declared unfit for work
e) Her GP should be contacted for further information on the number of exacerbations of COPD

QUESTION 3: LUNG FUNCTION

You see a gentleman who is a stonemason in whom health surveillance noted a restrictive lung function pattern.

With regard to the next step in his management:

a) He should be removed from work
b) He requires a chest X-ray
c) He requires a tuberculosis (TB) test
d) The risk assessment should be re-evaluated
e) He needs increased health surveillance

QUESTION 4: HEALTH SURVEILLANCE

You start work at a business where fettling is undertaken. The silica workplace exposure limit has been breached on risk assessment and you have been asked to formulate a health surveillance programme for workers.

a) Health surveillance is not a form of control
b) Health surveillance aims to limit disease severity
c) Workers and unions should be involved in the making of a health surveillance programme
d) Pre-employment screening and health screening are the same
e) Workers should be informed of what the results will be used for

QUESTION 5: RADIATION

You are undertaking a pre-employment health check on a 35-year-old lady about to start work as an industrial radiographer.

a) A history of previous radiotherapy is unlikely to make her unfit for work
b) A history of significant mental health illness should be determined
c) She must inform her employer at least verbally if she becomes pregnant
d) If she becomes pregnant she should wait until the viability has been established before informing her employer in writing
e) Because of the risk of blood dyscrasias when working with radiation, a baseline full blood count should be undertaken before she starts work

QUESTION 6: DISPUTES

You are undertaking health surveillance in a large car manufacturing firm when it becomes obvious that an employee is having symptoms of occupational asthma. You discuss this with him; he refuses to stop work and refuses consent for a report to be sent.

a) If he refuses to inform his employer then you should do so anyway, in his best interests
b) If he refuses to stop working despite knowing the risks of continuing then the employer has no duty of care towards him
c) He cannot continue to work in the same job despite his refusal to stop, and you should inform the employer that he is not fit to work
d) The minimum information that the employer can receive as a result of health surveillance is whether an employee is fit or unfit for work
e) You should increase his health surveillance

QUESTION 7: MENTAL HEALTH

A secondary school teacher has an episode of mania after which she reveals that she has a diagnosis of bipolar disorder. She tells you that she previously has not had an episode for 3 years. Her employer has told you that she voluntarily went off sick when she realised she was becoming unwell. She tells you that she has been taking her medication throughout and that her trigger for this event has now resolved. She tells you that she has been feeling well for 2 weeks. She tells you that she would like to return to work. She is happy for you to disclose all of your consultation to her employer.

a) Declare her unfit for work for a few more weeks, to ensure that this episode is over
b) Declare her condition to her employer and state that this means that she will be unfit for work for the foreseeable future
c) Declare her fit for work, disclose her condition and suggest that a wellness recovery action plan is put in place
d) Declare her unfit for work and write to her psychiatrist to confirm her condition and confirm her diagnosis and her compliance before allowing her back to work
e) Declare her fit for work, and, as you feel that the Equality Act applies, suggest that she be allowed time off to attend any medical appointments that she has, related to this condition

QUESTION 8: FITNESS TO ATTEND MEETINGS

You see a lady who has been signed off her work as a children's nursery worker. She has had many sporadic absences from work and as a result is on a final warning disciplinary. She has been signed off work for the last 2 weeks as a result of being presented with this disciplinary, with a diagnosis from the GP of 'work-related stress'; she tells you that she is increasingly anxious about the thought of having to undertake a meeting with management. She tells you that she feels low but denies any suicidal thoughts or self-harm. She cries at the thought of attending the meeting. She has a past history of depression.

Regarding your opinion on her ability to attend the meeting:

a) State in your report that she is not fit to attend the meeting at this point, and that it should go ahead without her
b) Try to persuade her to attend the meeting
c) State in your report that she is fit to attend a meeting about her absence
d) State In your report that her sporadic absences are likely to do with her depression and should be taken into account
e) Suggest adjustments to help her attend the meeting

QUESTION 9: CHRONIC FATIGUE SYNDROME

You see a 42-year-old teaching assistant with chronic fatigue syndrome. She tells you that she is not on any medication for her chronic fatigue. You are concerned about this. Her employer is willing to fund her therapy.

Regarding management for her, the most appropriate would be:

a) Graded exercise therapy
b) Counselling
c) Amitriptyline
d) Sertraline
e) Pain management

QUESTION 10: VIBRATION

Regarding the safe level of vibration exposure:

a) There is no safe level of vibration
b) Under 2.5 m/s² A(8)
c) Under 5 m/s² A(8)
d) 100 points
e) Under 400 points

QUESTION 11: HAND ARM VIBRATION SYNDROME (HAVS)

You see a stonemason who reports tingling of his fingers. He works with vibrating tools for most of the day. His symptoms are worse at night and on examination he has no blanching of his fingers. Tinel's is positive. He does not display symptoms on raising his arms.

a) You recommend that he should be prescribed nifedipine
b) Those with Raynaud's should not be working with vibrating tools
c) HAVS is not the only RIDDOR reportable disease related to vibration
d) A cervical rib is a possible differential diagnosis of HAVS
e) You should undertake a workplace inspection

QUESTION 12: HIERARCHY OF CONTROL

You are approached by a medical student who is learning about occupational health. He has seen a case of Hand Arm Vibration Syndrome in a dockyard worker. He has undertaken a risk assessment and wants some advice on control after a risk assessment.

The best form of control he can undertake is:

a) Health surveillance
b) Vibration-reducing gloves
c) Maintaining equipment
d) Job rotation
e) Allowing the operators to pick their own tools

QUESTION 13: HAND ARM VIBRATION SYNDROME (HAVS)

You see a gentleman whom you diagnose as having HAVS on health surveillance.

Regarding the most relevant information his employer needs to know:

a) Severe HAVS is RIDDOR reportable
b) He can no longer work with vibrating tools as he has a diagnosis of HAVS
c) He is entitled to industrial injuries disablement benefit
d) He can reduce the exacerbation of symptoms with gloves
e) A risk assessment needs to be carried out

QUESTION 14: HAND ARM VIBRATION SYNDROME (HAVS)

You evaluate a HAVS risk assessment in a dockyard. The workers on the pneumatic drills are at an exposure action value of 2.4 m/s^2 A(8). The employer would like to reduce the risk problems due to the effects of vibrations. There have been no reported vibration-related problems in his workforce.

Regarding reducing the levels of vibration:

a) No action is needed as HAVS does not occur below 2.5 m/s^2 A(8)
b) Reduce the length of time the employee uses the machine
c) Reduce the frequency of vibrations of the machine
d) Double the distance from the machine
e) Health surveillance is needed at this level of vibration

QUESTION 15: HEATWAVE

It has been a hot summer. Workers on a production line are complaining that their personal protective equipment (PPE) is making them unbearably warm. You are asked to provide advice on avoiding heat stress in a heatwave. Management are keen to avoid reduction in margins.

a) Workers do not have to wear their PPE in a heatwave as the risk of overheating is too high
b) Workers should be allowed to work at a slower pace
c) Workers should be allowed to rotate out of this environment more frequently
d) Alternative lightweight PPE should be considered
e) Workers should be allowed to go home

QUESTION 16: OCCUPATIONAL ASTHMA

Mr Taleb is a 37-year-old baker who has been asked to see you after his annual occupational spirometry which has showed a reversible obstructive lung function. He tells you that he gets a wheeze which is better during his holidays. He has a history of childhood asthma and is an ex-smoker of 20 pack years.

a) Mr Taleb is likely to have occupational asthma and should be put on restricted duties effective immediately
b) This employee is likely to have occupational asthma and respiratory PPE is therefore needed for all workers
c) Mr Taleb is likely to have occupational asthma and needs repeat spirometry in 3 months to see if worsening
d) Mr Taleb is likely to have occupational asthma and needs serial peak flows
e) This employee is likely to have occupational asthma and therefore health surveillance of all workers is needed

QUESTION 17: HEALTH SURVEILLANCE

You are asked to see a newly qualified hairdresser who refuses to take part in her contracted responsibility to undertake health surveillance. She says that she does not undertake much wet work and so does not think that she needs to take part in surveillance.

a) The employee has a right not to take part at her own risk and no further involvement from occupational health is needed
b) Management may have a right to terminate her contract
c) As long as she is following the wet work policy she does not need health surveillance as she should not be at risk
d) Health surveillance aims to protect the worker and detect pathology at the earliest incidence to minimise risk
e) This employee must be redeployed if she refuses to take part in health surveillance

QUESTION 18: HEARING LOSS

Ms Singh is an employee with noise-related hearing loss, found on health surveillance. She works with noisy pneumatic drills. You need to establish what information would be useful in investigating whether this is a work-related pathology.

a) Exploration of her hobbies
b) Whether she has been wearing her ear defenders
c) Pre-employment audiology
d) Whether she is going to make a claim
e) Past gentamicin use

QUESTION 19: ASBESTOS

Ms Lorrell is a contractor working on a relatively new building as a carpenter. After she undertook a risk assessment and commenced work, a small amount of asbestos was found in the walls unexpectedly.

a) Work should stop immediately and a risk assessment should be undertaken
b) Work should stop immediately until it is established whether all the contractors have asbestos training
c) Work should stop and all of those potentially exposed should have chest X-rays
d) Work should stop and the incident be reported by RIDDOR
e) Work should stop until all are provided with personal protective equipment

QUESTION 20: CHEST PAIN

Mr Singh is a 67-year-old truck loader who has been asked to see you a year after a failed stent following a myocardial infarction. He is on maximal medication. Recent correspondence from his cardiologist states that he is not fit for any further interventions. He is currently on light duties. He tells you that he continues to have chest pain on minimal exertion and at times of stress and uses his glyceryl trinitrate spray "nearly every day", including today.

a) This patient is likely to be temporarily unfit for his role with immediate effect; you should send him home
b) You should get a specialist opinion from a cardiologist before making a decision on Mr Singh's fitness for work
c) This patient is permanently unfit for his role and should be transferred to a sedentary role with immediate effect
d) This patient is temporarily unfit for work and should be transferred into a sedentary role immediately
e) It is your medical opinion and decision that Mr Singh is not capable for his contracted role and that his contract should be terminated if his angina is not well controlled after a set period of time

QUESTION 21: EPILEPSY

You are asked to review a contracting handyman who works on multiple sites. He is attending for pre-employment screening as he is being taken on as a permanent employee. He has been seen by the occupational health nurse who has stated that due to his epilepsy he should not work alone or at heights. He has not had a fit in 2 years and is on medication. It comes to light that he drives a van for work.

a) The employer should confirm that he is fit to drive his vehicle
b) He should not work at heights due to his risk of epilepsy
c) He cannot drive a Group 2 vehicle with his condition
d) You should write to his GP to confirm his last fit
e) He is fit for work with no restrictions

QUESTION 22: REPORTS

You are writing a report for an employer who wants to know whether an employee, Ms Penn, falls under the Equality Act 2010. Ms Penn has arthritis affecting both hips, limiting her ability to work as a marine biologist. She also has a past history of mild atrial fibrillation.

Regarding your assessment of the application of the Equality Act:

a) The ultimate decision is made by the Chairman of the Employment Tribunal rather than the medical profession, and therefore you cannot give an opinion
b) She definitely qualifies as disabled under the Equality Act 2010
c) Activities of daily living include breathing and eliminating waste
d) Getting out of a chair could be considered part of a functional assessment
e) If she has a disability Blue Badge for parking, she will fall under the Equality Act 2010

QUESTION 23: BLOOD-BORNE VIRUS

You are asked to review a pre-employment questionnaire. Mr Johanssen is a nurse who has disclosed that he is hepatitis B positive. He does not attend for his consultation.

a) Write to his hepatologist to gain information on his infectivity status, as this is relevant to his fitness for work
b) He can work as a nurse with hepatitis B and therefore you should confirm with his employer that he is fit to work with this disease
c) You need to gain his consent before communicating with his employer or doctors
d) He cannot work as a nurse with hepatitis B
e) He needs to be seen in order to find out how he acquired the disease

QUESTION 24: STATISTICS

You are teaching a medical student at a quarrying company where screening test A is used as part of a surveillance programme.

Test A gives the following results:

Test Result		DISEASE PRESENCE	
		+	−
	+	80	10
	−	20	90

Regarding test A's application as a screening tool:

a) The sensitivity of test A is 0.9
b) The sensitivity is used to detect the presence of disease
c) A sensitivity and specificity of 1 is desirable
d) Test A is a poor screening tool
e) A high specificity is needed for a good screening test

QUESTION 25: LUNG FUNCTION

You are given a spirometry result for Mr Ted, a 50-year-old gentleman who has worked as a tree surgeon for 25 years. The result shows an FEV of 70% and an FEV/FEVC ratio of 60%.

The most likely cause of his result is:

a) Tobacco
b) Crocidolite
c) Silica
d) Idiopathic
e) Isocyanates

QUESTION 26: ASTHMA

Mrs Giani works as a baker. After extensive peak flows, you provisionally diagnose her with occupational asthma after a year in the bakery.

a) You should undertake IgE tests to confirm the diagnosis
b) Refer her to a respiratory consultant for further management
c) You should advise the employee that redeployment will be necessary
d) Management should be informed that the employee's prognosis is poor
e) You should inform Mrs Giani that her smoking history may have contributed to her condition

QUESTION 27: LATEX

You see a 32-year-old lady who has just been diagnosed with a type I latex allergy.

With regard to her continuing to work:

a) She needs to be redeployed
b) Switching to powder-free gloves would not help
c) It will not make any clinical difference if her colleagues switch to low protein gloves
d) Respiratory personal protective equipment (PPE) may be needed
e) Immunotherapy may be needed

QUESTION 28: PREGNANCY

You see a 32-year-old nurse who is 13 weeks pregnant. So far the pregnancy has been uncomplicated and she is well. She has just told her employer and has been referred to you as a result, as she tells you that she wishes not to work nights – she fears it may harm the baby. However, her employer has not changed her contract.

a) Pregnancy falls under the Equality Act and therefore she is entitled to reasonable adjustments
b) The employer must undertake a new risk assessment of her role, as she is pregnant
c) Elimination of night shifts may not be a reasonable adjustment
d) Pregnancy is not an illness and so does not fall under the Equality Act
e) A reduction in prolonged standing may be considered a reasonable adjustment

QUESTION 29: CONSENT

You see 45-year-old postman. He has been referred to Occupational Health because he has breached the absence threshold and it is the employer's policy to refer at this point. The referral states that he has multiple 1- or 2-day absences with 'viral illnesses'. He tells you in confidence that he has depression and is taking time off for counselling and on days when his motivation is low. He tells you that he does not want to lose his job and does not want a report to go to his employer. Despite your best efforts he will not give his consent for a report to be released.

a) The Occupational Health practitioner has a contract with the employer that obliges them to send a report, otherwise they are in breach of contract
b) He is not demonstrating capacity and therefore his refusal of consent is not valid
c) You should advise him that his reluctance to allow information for a report suggests that he is deliberately misinforming his employer
d) Without relevant information the employer can act on the information they have
e) You can write a letter to state that the employee has refused consent

QUESTION 30: REPORTS

You see a 56-year-old gentleman who works as a heavy goods vehicle (HGV) driver. He has been absent from work with bilateral knee and hip osteoarthritis for 6 months and has been referred to you for the first time, as management are concerned about the length of time he has had off work. He claims that he cannot climb in and out of the HGV. He is still driving a car and tells you that he can undertake the emergency stop procedure in both vehicles. He tells you that he is awaiting an arthroscopy of his right knee. On examination, the range of movement of his knee is moderately limited bilaterally with bilateral crepitus and he has a mildly antalgic gait.

a) You should suggest that his paid sick leave be extended as a reasonable adjustment
b) You should seek further information on his management from his treating doctor
c) You should advise that he is fit to attend a meeting regarding his sickness absence
d) You should advise that he is unfit for the foreseeable future
e) You should advise that he cannot be fired because he falls under the Equality Act 2010

QUESTION 31: BACK PAIN

You see a 20-year-old man who works as a carpenter in the boat-making industry. He is complaining of a twisting back injury after tripping 2 weeks ago. He has been off sick with back pain ever since. He has no red flags in his history, and on examination he has no neurology and a reasonable range of movement.

Regarding his return to work:

a) An accident analysis should be undertaken
b) He could return to work despite pain
c) A lumbar support would be useful
d) There is good evidence that light duties help to resolve back pain
e) A phased return is needed

QUESTION 32: DVLA

You see a 30-year-old student who had a witnessed loss of consciousness whilst sitting at his desk. The witness reportedly told him that he came around after a few seconds and he denies any prodromal symptoms and tells you that he was fully aware of himself and his surroundings when he regained consciousness. You look at the DVLA guidelines that state that he should not drive for one month and that he should inform the DVLA. He is adamant that it will not happen again and states that he will not drive if it happens again.

a) You should take his car keys away from him
b) Inform him that he will be fined by the DVLA if he is caught driving
c) You should let him know that he is entitled to a second opinion
d) Tell him that under no circumstances can he drive at present
e) Consult with a medical protection advisor before you inform the DVLA

QUESTION 33: ACCESS TO MEDICAL RECORDS ACT

You discuss the outline of your report with an employee who wishes to see a copy of the report before it is sent to the employer.

a) The Access to Medical Records Act 1998 (AMRA) does not apply to occupational health physicians
b) The patient has 21 days under the AMRA to view the report and consent to its release
c) General Medical Council (GMC) guidance suggests that the patient should be allowed to see the report prior to the employer
d) All patients should be given the opportunity to see the report before their employer
e) The report cannot be released without the employee's consent under any circumstance unless there is a risk to public safety, the safety of others, or regarding an infectious disease.

QUESTION 34: MENOPAUSE

You see a 54-year-old lady who has been referred after it was brought to management's attention that she was very irritable. She denied any problems with work or at home and any medical problems to management as part of a review because of this. Human Resources (HR) is asking you whether there is any medical problem to account for her behaviour and to advise if so on going forward to support her at work. She works as a receptionist in a busy hotel.

When you consult with her she tells you that she is going through the menopause and that she has been struggling with mood swings and difficulty sleeping for 2 months. She tells you that she did not want to discuss this with her line manager.

She consents for your report to be sent to her employer.

a) You should advise HR that she is menopausal
b) You should advise HR that there is no medical problem underlying her behaviour
c) You should advise HR that shift changes may be appropriate to help with sleeping difficulties
d) You should advise HR that she should have reasonable adjustments
e) You should advise HR that the Equality Act is not likely to apply

QUESTION 35: DVLA

You see a driver of an 8-seater vehicle who had a stroke one month ago. He has no neurological deficit and is driving his car with no problem.

The employer has asked to know if he is fit to drive at work.

a) It is the employer's responsibility to contact the DVLA to confirm that the driver's licence is no longer rescinded
b) As long as he has no neurological deficit he can drive an 8-seater vehicle
c) Within the DVLA guidelines he is not fit to drive a Group 2 vehicle
d) You should ensure that he does not undertake any heavy lifting
e) If you are unsure, you should contact the DVLA for advice

QUESTION 36: SHINGLES

You see a 60-year-old personal assistant to the chief executive of an advertising company who was diagnosed one week ago with shingles on her abdomen.

Work had insisted that she stays off work for one week, and also that she sees occupational health for advice before she can return to work.

a) Employees should be advised that she has shingles
b) She can return to work with no restrictions
c) Pregnant employees working with her should be tested for immunity
d) Other employees in her department do not routinely need to have the chickenpox vaccination
e) She should not be in contact with the general public in case they have low immunity

QUESTION 37: CHICKENPOX

You are asked to see a 30-year-old bank Health Care Assistant who has come into contact with a patient two days before they developed disseminated shingles. She says that she has not had chickenpox. She is asymptomatic but worried.

a) She is not likely to contract the disease because she was in contact with the patient outside of the incubation period
b) Her occupational health notes should show her immunisation status
c) If she develops symptoms she should be excluded from work
d) Varicella zoster virus immunoglobulin should routinely be offered to vulnerable healthcare workers
e) She is within the incubation period. Generally hospital pre-employment checks will include immunity status. She may be immune, and if not then varicella zoster virus immunoglobulin should routinely be offered to vulnerable healthcare workers

QUESTION 38: UPPER LIMB DISORDERS

Mr Dale is a 24-year-old picker in a toy warehouse. For the last 3 months he tells you that he has had pain in his right forearm and elbow. He is left-handed. In his spare time he plays darts, but has not been able to do so because of the pain. He is otherwise fit and well. On abduction of the elbow against resistance he complains of pain. You know that other packers have similar symptoms and suspect that the organisation needs to undertake a risk assessment.

a) Risk should not be assessed using a questionnaire
b) Training is a form of control
c) There are no legal provisions specific to work-related upper limb disorders
d) Assessing neck pain is appropriate
e) Employees and safety advisors should be involved in preventative measures

QUESTION 39: DIABETES

You are asked to see a district nurse to advise on any adjustments needed to her work as a result of her ongoing pregnancy. She is 30/40. She has gestational diabetes and has been started on insulin one month ago, with no complications so far. She is otherwise well and her blood sugars have been stable. Driving is integral to her role.

Regarding advice you should give her and her employer:

a) An adjustment to be considered would be a driver/escort as she legally cannot drive without DVLA clearance
b) She does not need to inform the DVLA of her diabetes
c) If she can show that her insulin levels have been stable for one month then she can drive
d) Her employer must undertake a risk assessment now that she is pregnant
e) She should be restricted from lone working because of the risk of hypoglycaemia

QUESTION 40: DIABETES

You are asked to see a poorly controlled type 2 diabetic who is a trainee paramedic, for an opinion on fitness for her role. She is not on insulin, but tells you that her consultant has advised her that she may need to be 'in the future'.

a) She cannot drive an ambulance if she is medicated with insulin, regardless of her glycaemic control
b) She will be subject to yearly DVLA checks to confirm her fitness to drive an ambulance
c) She should not undertake night shift work until her glycaemic control is established
d) She will need to wear a continuous glucose monitor to reduce the risk of hypoglycaemia in an emergency situation
e) She needs to ensure her HbA1c is less than 70 to be able to drive an ambulance

QUESTION 41: NEEDLE-STICK INJURIES

You consult with a frantic junior doctor who has just obtained a needle-stick injury from a patient in A and E. The donor has just died.

The next line of management by occupational health would be to:

a) Take blood from the donor
b) Start post-exposure prophylaxis
c) Report the incident to RIDDOR
d) Undertake an accident analysis
e) Suggest a restriction from exposure-prone procedures

QUESTION 42: ALCOHOL

You are in clinic when a junior doctor asks for some urgent advice. She thinks that her consultant is drunk because he is acting oddly and she smelt alcohol on his breath.

She does not know what to do.

a) The consultant is not fit for work, with immediate effect
b) Advise her to bring him to the occupational health department for immediate testing
c) He should be referred to occupational health for a review
d) Give her an Alcoholics Anonymous leaflet to give to him
e) She must inform the consultant's line manager immediately

QUESTION 43: UPPER LIMB DISORDERS

You see a 35-year-old administrator who complains of pain in her right elbow which is worse on most movements and appears to be aggravated by long periods of time typing on the computer. She is able to undertake activities outside of work, but finds that after an hour of being at work her symptoms get worse. She tells you that she has tried wrist splints, non-steroidal anti-inflammatory drugs (NSAIDs) and physiotherapy, and is keen to have any other suggestions.

a) There is no specific legislation directly related to upper limb disorders
b) The Health and Safety Executive specifies 15-minute breaks every 3 hours for employees with upper limb disorders
c) Vibration can make upper limb disorders worse
d) The employer has a duty to provide job enlargement
e) Yellow flags are an indicator of poor prognosis

QUESTION 44: HOME WORKING

You see a 45-year-old data manager who is recovering from chemotherapy. As part of his return to work plan he has requested to work at home for 2 days a week. The employer has approved this request.

a) Employers do not have a duty of care to employees who work from home
b) Employers have a duty to apply the same health and safety standards to home workers as those in the workplace
c) A risk assessment can be undertaken by the employee
d) The employer is only responsible for ensuring the electrical safety of the equipment that they provide
e) The health and safety of others in the home should be considered in the risk assessment

QUESTION 45: MENTAL HEALTH

You see a carpenter in a large construction site who tells you that he is feeling low. He tells you that 2 months ago he tried to commit suicide by hanging himself, but was found by his girlfriend. He tells you that he has been at work since this event (work are not aware of it) and that he is being followed up by the crisis team once a week. He tells you that as far as he is aware, there are no concerns from management about the quality of his work. His role involves working at height, working alone, and working with moving part machinery.

Regarding the next management step to take:

a) He is not fit for work
b) He should not undertake lone working
c) He should undertake a Wellness Recovery Plan with management
d) He should increase his medication
e) You should write to his psychiatrist to determine his suicide risk

QUESTION 46: HUMAN IMMUNODEFICIENCY VIRUS (HIV)

You undertake a pre-employment consultation with Mr Bleasdale, a 32-year-old man applying for a role at Maydie Hospital as a porter. He discloses that he is HIV positive, with a CD4 count over 400, and no other medical problems. At present he is not on antiviral therapy due to problems with unacceptable side-effects, but is due to see his consultant for a review of medications in 2 months. He has a past history of carpal tunnel syndrome, for which he wears splints at night, and has a history of epilepsy. He is on 500 mg of Keppra, and his last fit was 2 months ago, when he had three fits in one week.

Regarding what you should inform Human Resources of:

a) He is unfit for role
b) He is fit with restrictions: he should not enter the chemotherapy ward
c) He is fit for role with no restrictions
d) He can work in a hospital environment with a diagnosis of HIV
e) He should not undertake lone working

QUESTION 47: CARDIOLOGY

An employee has cardiac trouble and has a pacemaker fitted, then returns unannounced, appearing on site back at work one day where electromagnetic fields are present. The manager both phones and emails you in a panic, asking if the individual is fit for work and whether or not they can stay on site; are they fit for work and can they stay on site?

a) State that he is not fit and must leave the site immediately
b) Restrict his duties temporarily, with immediate effect
c) Place him on medical suspension until you can obtain the answer
d) Advise that the Health and Safety Manager should make the decision
e) Write to the cardiologist and ask their opinion

QUESTION 48: DIABETES

A type 2 diabetic taxi driver has been referred to you for advice regarding fitness to drive and depression, and when you ask him about his medication he mentions that he was started on insulin 2 months ago for his diabetes.

Regarding his driving:

a) He needs to meet the Group 1 DVLA vehicle standards for diabetics, in order to be able to drive a taxi

b) Insurers can charge more for a diabetic driver's insurance only if there is evidence of increased risk

c) He needs to inform the DVLA otherwise his insurance could be invalidated

d) His ability to drive in the future will be subject to a yearly assessment by a consultant in diabetic medicine

e) If he wears a continuous blood glucose monitor, this would eliminate the need for specific blood glucose self-monitoring before driving

QUESTION 49: ILL HEALTH RETIREMENT

You see a 45-year-old teaching assistant who has applied for ill heath retirement. She tells you that she has arthritis of her left hip and is finding mobilising around a classroom and between classrooms painful. She describes her walking as slow, and feels that she does not want to disadvantage the children she helps by leaving the classroom early to get to her next class, but if she does not do this then she feels unable to walk fast enough to get to her next lesson on time. She comes with a supporting letter from her head teacher, which states that he is unable to accommodate any reduction in hours or change her working schedule so that her classes are closer together, nor can he provide a wheelchair; he feels that she needs ill health retirement as she clearly cannot work in her condition, and as a valued member of staff would have to be made redundant. On examination she walks with a three wheeler aid, is very slow to mobilise, has difficulty getting in and out of a chair, and is morbidly obese.

a) You should declare her suitable for ill health retirement due to poor mobility
b) You should declare her not suitable for ill health retirement as it is likely that she could do other work
c) You should suggest that weight reduction could enable her to work
d) Declare her unfit for work for the foreseeable future due to arthritis
e) Suggest she is fit for work at another school which does not have access limitations

QUESTION 50: BACK PAIN

You see a 34-year-old carpenter who suffers from recurrent low back pain. He has no red flag symptoms or signs. His examination is limited by pain. He does not take any analgesia as he 'does not like to take medication'. He tells you that this episode was exacerbated by a work episode where he had to lift a heavy door by himself. You have noticed an increasing incidence of back pain in workers in his department.

a) An ergonomics assessment takes into account organisational factors
b) The employee requires a manual handling refresher
c) The Assessment of Repetitive Tasks tool should be used to assess employee risk
d) Lifting from a paraneutral position will aid appropriate lifting
e) Preventative measures can be cost-effective

QUESTION 51: SAFEGUARDING

You see a sales assistant who has been referred with depression. She is a single mum and looks unkempt. You think that she has severe depression. On her way out, you notice that she has left her 2-year-old daughter on her own in the waiting room. You observe that the girl looks malnourished and dirty and you feel there is the potential that she has been neglected.

a) A referral to social services for support can be made without consent
b) A referral to social services for safeguarding issues can be made without consent
c) A referral to social services for support needs consent
d) The best action is to speak to the employer
e) If a client discloses their own abuse towards their child they should be encouraged to tell the police

QUESTION 52: PRE-EMPLOYMENT SCREENING

Ms Smith has applied for job as an administrator on an obstetric ward. She has refused a complete screening test to check her varicella zoster virus status and declares that she has not had chickenpox.

a) Check that she has been properly informed as to why the test is needed
b) The Occupational Health Physician has a duty of care towards the employee in this instance
c) An employer cannot be obliged to undertake the risk of employing her
d) The Occupational Health Physician should write to the GP for her medical records
e) She is a risk to the unborn child

QUESTION 53: BIOLOGICAL MONITORING

Regarding biological monitoring:

a) Consent is always needed to take samples for monitoring
b) Ill health is not likely to occur at levels exceeding the benchmark value
c) An occupational nurse can be used for the interpretation of the results
d) An occupational physician can be used to collect the samples
e) Ill health is not likely to occur at values above the health guidance value

QUESTION 54: HAND ARM VIBRATION SYNDROME (HAVS)

A 30-year-old shipbuilder presents with intermittent tingling and blanching in his left hand. He works with many vibrating tools. He has a family history of systemic lupus erythematosus (his mum). He has a marked left-sided tremor (in his left hand only). He has reduced power globally in his left forearm. Fine motor movements were normal. Purdue test was normal and monofilament tests were normal also. Phalen's and Tinel's are unremarkable.

Regarding the next option in managing this employee:

a) Advise a GP review
b) Refer for a tier 5 HAVS assessment
c) Ask management to provide a vibration risk assessment
d) Advise more frequent health surveillance
e) Advise the employee to provide proof of hand blanching

QUESTION 55: MISCELLANEOUS

You see a professor of physics who has been referred after complaining of 'exhaustion'. She tells you that she has just finished a project that she has found challenging and has also had to manage two colleagues who have not been getting on.

She denies that she is 'stressed'. She tells you that she has had reduced sleep but no other symptoms.

Her employer wants advice regarding the best way of avoiding a relapse of her symptoms.

a) There is no way of controlling her symptoms as no problems have been identified
b) Exhaustion can be caused by medical problems such as hypothyroidism and she should see her GP for blood tests
c) Reducing job demands could help
d) Increasing her control over her work could reduce the likelihood of the development of work-related stress
e) A work stress risk assessment is appropriate to help identify triggers

QUESTION 56: TOURETTE'S SYNDROME

You see a 35-year-old lecturer with Tourette's syndrome. He is facing a disciplinary for offensive behaviour, as there have been several complaints about comments he has made (possibly as part of his syndrome); as part of a management plan has been referred to occupational health.

Regarding the advice you should give:

a) He is likely to fall under the Equality Act 2010
b) Controlling his outbursts is a management issue
c) Lorazepam could be used to control these outbursts
d) His students and colleagues should be made aware of his condition, to reduce complaints
e) It is not appropriate for him to be teaching

QUESTION 57: UPPER LIMB DISORDERS

You see an administrator who complains of pain and numbness in the thumb and first finger of her right hand. She thinks that her symptoms only occur at work whilst she is typing. A workstation assessment has been undertaken before she sees you, but she tells you that a split keyboard and penguin mouse have not helped. She feels that her symptoms are getting worse. Tinel's and Phalen's tests are negative. She is becoming less productive and management are keen to know what help may be available for her.

a) Advise a course of non-steroidal anti-inflammatory drugs
b) Referral to occupational therapist
c) Request the GP to refer for nerve conduction tests
d) Write to the GP to request a referral to a hand surgeon
e) Advise the patient to seek a steroid injection

QUESTION 58: BLUE LIGHT DRIVING

You have seen a stable insulin-dependent diabetic policewoman with an HbA1c of 65. She has had a car accident where the matter of her fitness to drive police vehicles is being questioned.

a) She can drive an unmarked police car
b) She can drive a blue light vehicle
c) She cannot drive a blue light vehicle in any circumstance due to the risk of hypoglycaemia
d) An individual decision can be made at the discretion of the Force Medical Adviser
e) Refer to the DVLA guidelines

QUESTION 59: EPILEPSY

Regarding the maximum level of annual risk of sustaining a seizure accepted for holding a Group 2 driving licence:

a) 2%
b) <2%
c) 4%
d) <4%
e) 20%

QUESTION 60: NOISE

Health and Safety perform a risk assessment of a factory and identify that the noise levels are too high.

Regarding the most appropriate form of control:

a) Anti-vibration mounting under machinery
b) Reduction of the amount of time employees are using the machinery
c) Constructive interference/superposition
d) Ear defenders
e) Health surveillance

ANSWERS to Mock exam

QUESTION 1: ANOREXIA

You see a 20-year-old girl whose fitness to undertake a teaching degree you have been asked to assess. She has a past history of anorexia, and was admitted against her will into an eating disorders clinic 2 years ago. She tells you that she left of her own accord after 2 weeks. She tells you that since then she has completed her Duke of Edinburgh Gold Award and has been feeling well. She denies any ongoing problems. She looks to be of a normal BMI. She refuses to be weighed. She appears enthusiastic about her course.

The answer is: a) You should declare her unfit for her role

It is clear from her desire not to be weighed, combined with the recent history of declared active and serious health condition and refusal to engage in services, that there is a strong possibility that she has not recovered, despite what she is saying.

A GP report would not provide objective information on her compliance since leaving hospital, nor on concurrent health issues, BMI trend and her insight into her condition. She is unlikely to attend her GP, let them weigh her, or discuss matters frankly.

An objective psychiatrist's review is a potential next step but this will not give us any information into how severe her disease was, nor when it occurred.

Teachers need to have the health and wellbeing necessary to deal with the specific types of teaching problems and associated duties (adjusted, as appropriate) in which they are engaged (fitness to teach guidelines).

QUESTION 2: CHRONIC OBSTRUCTIVE PULMONARY DISEASE (COPD)

You see a 67-year-old lunchtime and playground supervisor with COPD applying for ill health retirement. She currently works 7 hours a week at a primary school. Her job involves handing out school meals and supervising the children whilst they eat, for one hour a day. She has an exercise tolerance of 20 metres "on a good day" but declares no exacerbations in the last 2 years. She is not on any oxygen but is on maximal other medical therapies, which is confirmed by the respiratory specialist's letter confirming stage 4 COPD and a FEV_1 of <30%. She tells you that she has no other skills to be able to do another job.

The criteria for ill health retirement require fulfilment of the following:

1) She has an infirmity of body or mind rendering her unable to do her contractual role;
2) She is not immediately fit for other gainful employment due to ill health for 12 consecutive months.

The answer is: b) This lady meets the criteria for ill health retirement

With an exercise tolerance of 20 m it is unlikely the LTOT/mobile oxygen will help with her symptoms to the point that she would be able to walk around a playground, for example. Therefore writing to her specialist would be unlikely to tell you any new information; neither would knowing the number of exacerbations she has had. She may be fit to do a sedentary role in theory on medical grounds; her skill mix does not determine this, instead it is the medical status. Stage 4 COPD has a very poor one-year prognosis and she may not live for 12 months. She is indeed unfit for her role, but this is not the best answer, given she has applied for ill health retirement.

She has stage 4 COPD, which NICE describes as "very severe". This is end stage disease with a 4-year survival rate of <20% (NICE, 2011, CG101).

NICE, CG101: *Chronic obstructive pulmonary disease in over 16s: diagnosis and management* (2010).

https://cks.nice.org.uk/chronic-obstructive-pulmonary-disease#!scenario:2 states: "End-stage chronic obstructive pulmonary disease (COPD) should be suspected when COPD is very severe (forced expiratory volume in 1 second [FEV_1] less than 30% predicted, and/or Medical Research Council [MRC] dyspnoea scale grade 4 or 5) and is both unresponsive to medical treatment, and associated with a probable life expectancy of less than 6–12 months."

QUESTION 3: LUNG FUNCTION

You see a gentleman who is a stonemason in whom health surveillance noted a restrictive lung function pattern.

With regard to the next step in his management:

The answer is: b) He requires a chest X-ray

Note the question asks about the next step in his management – therefore whilst the controls should be looked at if an employee appears to be presenting with an occupational disease, this would not be the best answer. He should firstly have a chest X-ray to determine the cause of the restrictive pattern – it may not be a pneumoconiosis at all! A TB test is not necessary unless he has other symptoms suggesting TB – pneumoconiosis is a risk factor for TB. Now that he has reduced lung function he will need increased health surveillance.

QUESTION 4: HEALTH SURVEILLANCE

You start work at a business where fettling is undertaken. The silica workplace exposure limit has been breached on risk assessment and you have been asked to formulate a health surveillance programme for workers.

The answer is: c) Workers and unions should be involved in the making of a health surveillance programme

The next step would be to ask workers and unions to be involved in this process and outline what the results would be used for, etc.

QUESTION 5: RADIATION

You are undertaking a pre-employment health check on a 35-year-old lady about to start work as an industrial radiographer.

The answer is: b) A history of significant mental health illness should be determined

A significant mental health history is relevant, as working with radiation involves self-discipline and mental stability; this may be affected by serious mental illness which is uncontrolled, such as a personality disorder.

QUESTION 6: DISPUTES

You are undertaking health surveillance in a large car manufacturing firm when it becomes obvious that an employee is having symptoms of occupational asthma. You discuss this with him; he refuses to stop work and refuses consent for a report to be sent.

The answer is: b) If he refuses to stop working despite knowing the risks of continuing then the employer has no duty of care towards him

There have been trials regarding a scenario such as this, and the bottom line is that he can continue to work at his own risk as long as he knows the risks, and if he refuses permission for a report to be released as a result of his health surveillance consultation, then you cannot do so.

QUESTION 7: MENTAL HEALTH

A secondary school teacher has an episode of mania after which she reveals that she has a diagnosis of bipolar disorder. She tells you that she previously has not had an episode for 3 years. Her employer has told you that she voluntarily went off sick when she realised she was becoming unwell. She tells you that she has been taking her medication throughout and that her trigger for this event has now resolved. She tells you that she has been feeling well for 2 weeks. She tells you that she would like to return to work. She is happy for you to disclose all of your consultation to her employer.

The answer is: d) Declare her unfit for work and write to her psychiatrist to confirm her condition and confirm her diagnosis and her compliance before allowing her back to work

The main points of this question are to:
* determine her insight into her condition, as this will be key to her continuing to work. Good insight is suggested by:
    - her compliance with medication
    - a recognition that she was unwell and actions taken to remove herself from work
* determine any markers of continuing or unstable ill health (there are none).

You then need to decide how to plan to keep her well on a return to work: a W(R)AP is a good option:

www.mind.org.uk/media/1593680/guide-to-waps.pdf

www.workingtogetherforrecovery.co.uk/Documents/Wellness%20Recovery%20
Action%20Plan.pdf

You can confirm her diagnosis once she is back in role.

QUESTION 8: FITNESS TO ATTEND MEETINGS

You see a lady who has been signed off her work as a children's nursery worker. She
has had many sporadic absences from work and as a result is on a final warning
disciplinary. She has been signed off work for the last 2 weeks as a result of being
presented with this disciplinary, with a diagnosis from the GP of 'work-related stress';
she tells you that she is increasingly anxious about the thought of having to undertake
a meeting with management. She tells you that she feels low but denies any suicidal
thoughts or self-harm. She cries at the thought of attending the meeting. She has a
past history of depression.

Regarding your opinion on her ability to attend the meeting:

**The answer is: c) State in your report that she is fit to attend a meeting about
her absence**

Attending the meeting is unlikely to make her potential mental health worse in this
scenario, and therefore she is fit to attend. It could be that her absences are related to
a re-emergence of her past mental health diagnosis, but nothing definitively suggests
this from the question. You could persuade her to attend but this is not relevant to the
question. Suggesting adjustments may be useful.

QUESTION 9: CHRONIC FATIGUE SYNDROME

You see a 42-year-old teaching assistant with chronic fatigue syndrome. She tells you
that she is not on any medication for her chronic fatigue. You are concerned about this.
Her employer is willing to fund her therapy.

Regarding management for her, the most appropriate would be:

The answer is: a) Graded exercise therapy

Whilst most of the answer options may be relevant, NICE suggests graded exercise
therapy or CBT (not counselling) as first-line therapies.

QUESTION 10: VIBRATION

Regarding the safe level of vibration exposure:

The answer is: a) There is no safe level of vibration

There is no safe level of exposure and therefore an exposure action value has been set.

Levels must be kept as low as reasonably practicable at any exposure value, but 2.5 m/s² A(8) is the exposure action value at which other measures must be put into place to protect workers. At all levels, information and training must be provided for workers.

QUESTION 11: HAND ARM VIBRATION SYNDROME (HAVS)

You see a stonemason who reports tingling of his fingers. He works with vibrating tools for most of the day. His symptoms are worse at night and on examination he has no blanching of his fingers. Tinel's is positive. He does not display symptoms on raising his arms.

The answer is: e) You should undertake a workplace inspection

This worker appears superficially to have carpal tunnel syndrome that could potentially be vibration related. Therefore the level of vibration that he has been exposed to needs to be assessed, and a workplace assessment is therefore the best option.

QUESTION 12: HIERARCHY OF CONTROL

You are approached by a medical student who is learning about occupational health. He has seen a case of Hand Arm Vibration Syndrome in a dockyard worker. He has undertaken a risk assessment and wants some advice on control after a risk assessment.

The best form of control he can undertake is:

The answer is: c) Maintaining equipment

Here, engineering controls are the highest form of control. It is also important to note that there is no effective PPE for vibration.

QUESTION 13: HAND ARM VIBRATION SYNDROME (HAVS)

You see a gentleman whom you diagnose as having HAVS on health surveillance.

Regarding the most relevant information his employer needs to know:

The answer is: e) A risk assessment needs to be carried out

All HAVS is RIDDOR reportable.

Once a new disease has been reported, controls need to be evaluated.

Not all employees with HAVS can claim industrial injuries disablement benefit.

QUESTION 14: HAND ARM VIBRATION SYNDROME (HAVS)

You evaluate a HAVS risk assessment in a dockyard. The workers on the pneumatic drills are at an exposure action value of 2.4 m/s^2 A(8). The employer would like to reduce the risk problems due to the effects of vibrations. There have been no reported vibration-related problems in his workforce.

Regarding reducing the levels of vibration:

The answer is: c) Reduce the frequency of vibrations of the machine

Lower frequency vibration is less harmful.

The general principle regarding vibration is that even below the recommended 'safe levels', exposure should be kept as low as reasonably practicable.

HAVS is a vascular, neurological and musculoskeletal problem that occurs as a result of working with vibrating tools.

Vibration is expressed as a sum of vectors, with the unit m/s^2 A(8).

An exposure value of 2.5 m/s^2 or 100 points is the exposure action value (EAV).

The EAV is not the value below which is considered safe (as no level is technically safe) but is the value at which, if likely to be exceeded, health surveillance should be undertaken.

The exposure limit value is 5 m/s^2 or 400 points.

Workers should not be exposed to this and if they are, immediate action needs to be taken to control/prevent exposure.

QUESTION 15: HEATWAVE

It has been a hot summer. Workers on a production line are complaining that their personal protective equipment (PPE) is making them unbearably warm. You are asked to provide advice on avoiding heat stress in a heatwave. Management are keen to avoid reduction in margins.

The answer is: c) Workers should be allowed to rotate out of this environment more frequently

HSE has good guidance on heat stress.

A risk assessment should be undertaken. The most effective control based on the hierarchy of control would be the administrative control – working at a slower pace or rotating workers more frequently; the option least likely to reduce profit margins would be to rotate workers.

QUESTION 16: OCCUPATIONAL ASTHMA

Mr Taleb is a 37-year-old baker who has been asked to see you after his annual occupational spirometry which has showed a reversible obstructive lung function. He tells you that he gets a wheeze which is better during his holidays. He has a history of childhood asthma and is an ex-smoker of 20 pack years.

The answer is: d) Mr Taleb is likely to have occupational asthma and needs serial peak flows

You do not have objective proof that this is occupational asthma as of yet, as you only have the employee's history. The BOHRF gold standard suggests that the worker should be provided with a 'peak flow meter and asked to note, while still exposed, the best of three readings at least four times a day (for 2 weeks), to include consecutive days at and away from work'.

Once a diagnosis is confirmed then symptoms of other workers should be investigated.

QUESTION 17: HEALTH SURVEILLANCE

You are asked to see a newly qualified hairdresser who refuses to take part in her contracted responsibility to undertake health surveillance. She says that she does not undertake much wet work and so does not think that she needs to take part in surveillance.

The answer is: b) Management may have a right to terminate her contract

It is essential that employers have a robust health surveillance policy, which has been agreed with employees. It should state clearly why the surveillance is required, what action will be considered in the event of the employee being unable to continue working with a specific hazard – for example, redeployment within the company to an alternative area of work – and the consequences of non-compliance with the policy. This may also include termination. If an employee refuses to take part in a health surveillance programme, the employer must explore their rationale for the decision and attempt to persuade them to reconsider their actions. If an employee continues to refuse the required assessments, the employer should exclude them from further hazard exposure, if possible.

QUESTION 18: HEARING LOSS

Ms Singh is an employee with noise-related hearing loss, found on health surveillance. She works with noisy pneumatic drills. You need to establish what information would be useful in investigating whether this is a work-related pathology.

The answer is: c) Pre-employment audiology

Going back to first principles, you need to determine whether she has long-standing hearing loss from before this employment.

Whilst video gaming and not wearing PPE may play a part, if the hearing loss predates the employment then this may suggest that it is not work-related.

QUESTION 19: ASBESTOS

Ms Lorrell is a contractor working on a relatively new building as a carpenter. After she undertook a risk assessment and commenced work, a small amount of asbestos was found in the walls unexpectedly.

The answer is: a) Work should stop immediately and a risk assessment should be undertaken

A risk assessment should be undertaken as the first step to decide on the likelihood and level of harm, for adequate controls to be put in place. Asbestos exposure is not RIDDOR reportable, only asbestos-related lung disease associated with at-risk occupations.

QUESTION 20: CHEST PAIN

Mr Singh is a 67-year-old truck loader who has been asked to see you a year after a failed stent following a myocardial infarction. He is on maximal medication. Recent correspondence from his cardiologist states that he is not fit for any further interventions. He is currently on light duties. He tells you that he continues to have chest pain on minimal exertion and at times of stress and uses his glyceryl trinitrate spray "nearly every day", including today.

The answer is: a) This patient is likely to be temporarily unfit for his role with immediate effect; you should send him home

This patient is still having angina despite treatment, has a failed stent and is unlikely to be fit for any manual handling role; therefore he should not be undertaking this work at present. His stent has failed and therefore his prognosis for his ability to undertake his contractual role is not good. It would be worth clarifying with his cardiologist whether any further intervention can be undertaken, and once his angina is under control he could be redeployed to a job with minimal stress and much lighter duties.

QUESTION 21: EPILEPSY

You are asked to review a contracting handyman who works on multiple sites. He is attending for pre-employment screening as he is being taken on as a permanent employee. He has been seen by the occupational health nurse who has stated that due to his epilepsy he should not work alone or at heights. He has not had a fit in 2 years and is on medication. It comes to light that he drives a van for work.

The answer is: e) He is fit for work with no restrictions

He has already been undertaking the job for some time as a contractor. Under the DVLA guidelines, as long as he is being truthful about his last fit, he is able to drive a Group 1 vehicle; a van is a Group 1 vehicle. The DVLA works on the premise that if a person with epilepsy fulfils their driving criteria, then the likelihood of having another fit is <20%. Therefore, working on this basis if his risk is enough to drive a vehicle then his risk is enough to work alone and also to work at height.

QUESTION 22: REPORTS

You are writing a report for an employer who wants to know whether an employee, Ms Penn, falls under the Equality Act 2010. Ms Penn has arthritis affecting both hips, limiting her ability to work as a marine biologist. She also has a past history of mild atrial fibrillation.

Regarding your assessment of the application of the Equality Act:

The answer is: d) Getting out of a chair could be considered part of a functional assessment

In order to assess her likely eligibility for the Equality Act 2010, you would base this on Ms Penn's symptoms and functional assessment. If her symptoms are mild and therefore do not affect her activities of daily living, as partly outlined in option (c), then she may not be eligible. Just because she has a disability Blue Badge does not mean that all her medical problems qualify her for reasonable adjustments. For example, she may fall under the Equality Act with regard to her arthritis but not her atrial fibrillation. You can give an opinion on what you think would be the legal application of the Equality Act with regard to an employee, but this would be an opinion only.

QUESTION 23: BLOOD-BORNE VIRUS

You are asked to review a pre-employment questionnaire. Mr Johanssen is a nurse who has disclosed that he is hepatitis B positive. He does not attend for his consultation.

The answer is: c) You need to gain his consent before communicating with his employer or doctors

Consent is needed to release this sensitive data to Mr Johanssen's employer; just because he has disclosed this on his pre-employment questionnaire does not mean that he has given consent for anyone else to see this information. He can possibly work as a nurse with hepatitis B depending upon his role, e.g. he probably could not be a theatre nurse. You may wish, with his consent, to enquire about his treatment as this may affect his infectivity if he has a needle-stick injury/accident.

QUESTION 24: STATISTICS

You are teaching a medical student at a quarrying company where screening test A is used as part of a surveillance programme.

Test A gives the following results:

Test Result	DISEASE PRESENCE		
		+	−
	+	80	10
	−	20	90

Regarding test A's application as a screening tool:

The answer is: b) The sensitivity is used to detect the presence of disease

The sensitivity is the proportion of positive results (i.e. where there is disease present) with a positive test result (i.e. it has picked up the disease). A screening test should have a high sensitivity therefore, in order to accurately pick up positive cases. A test with high specificity is used to rule the disease in, i.e. as a confirmatory test once it appears disease is present. In an ideal world, every test would have a sensitivity and specificity of one. However this is not the reality!

QUESTION 25: LUNG FUNCTION

You are given a spirometry result for Mr Ted, a 50-year-old gentleman who has worked as a tree surgeon for 25 years. The result shows an FEV of 70% and an FEV/FEVC ratio of 60%.

The most likely cause of his result is:

The answer is: a) Tobacco

This spirometry shows an obstructive lung pattern. He is unlikely to have been exposed to significant amounts of asbestos or isocyanates in his occupation or outside of work, and therefore tobacco exposure (don't forget that indirect exposure may have been high in the past) is the most likely source.

QUESTION 26: ASTHMA

Mrs Giani works as a baker. After extensive peak flows, you provisionally diagnose her with occupational asthma after a year in the bakery.

The answer is: c) You should advise the employee that redeployment will be necessary

Using the BOHRF guidelines on occupational asthma: if the diagnosis is clear-cut after lung tests, then no further investigation/referral is needed. Prognosis is generally poor but can be related to length of time exposed to the allergen, and so removal of the exposure (in this case, by redeployment) is the next step.

QUESTION 27: LATEX

You see a 32-year-old lady who has just been diagnosed with a type I latex allergy.

With regard to her continuing to work:

The answer is: d) Respiratory personal protective equipment (PPE) may be needed

Source: *Latex Allergy: occupational aspects of management* (RCP, 2008) Available at www.hse.gov.uk/healthservices/latex/allergyguide.pdf

By far the most important occupational risk factor for latex sensitisation is the use of powdered latex gloves, as they have a higher latex allergen content than powder-free gloves.

In employees who are latex allergic/sensitised, taking latex avoidance measures results in cessation or diminution of symptoms. Markers of sensitisation decrease regardless of whether co-workers continue to use powder-free low protein latex gloves or latex-free gloves.

If there remains a significant risk to highly sensitive latex-allergic employees, use of certain respiratory protective equipment can help in reducing inhalational exposure.

QUESTION 28: PREGNANCY

You see a 32-year-old nurse who is 13 weeks pregnant. So far the pregnancy has been uncomplicated and she is well. She has just told her employer and has been referred to you as a result, as she tells you that she wishes not to work nights – she fears it may harm the baby. However, her employer has not changed her contract.

The answer is: c) Elimination of night shifts may not be a reasonable adjustment

Sources:
- *Physical and shift work in pregnancy: occupational aspects of management* (RCP, 2009) Available at physical-and-shift-work-in-pregnancy-summary-leaflet-for-healthcare-professionals.pdf
- *New and Expectant Mothers who Work* (HSE, 2003) Available at www.hse.gov.uk/pubns/indg373.pdf
- *New and Expectant Mothers at Work: a guide for health professionals* (HSE, 2003) Available at www.aber.ac.uk/en/media/departmental/healthsafetyenvironment/indg373hp.pdf

The Equality Act covers more than just illnesses! It does include pregnancy. Therefore she would be entitled to reasonable adjustments potentially (making option A a possibility). However, what would be considered reasonable, especially so early in her pregnancy, is a moot point.

The FOM suggests that 'there is insufficient evidence of a risk to pregnant women to make recommendations to restrict shift work, including rotating shifts or night/evening work'; therefore it would not be a reasonable adjustment. It does suggest that 'employers should reduce standing for longer than three hours for pregnant workers where possible, particularly in late pregnancy'.

The employer should undertake a risk assessment for the job to cover women in all stages of pregnancy. Given the prevalence of pregnant nurses, this is likely to have been done for a similar circumstance and therefore is unlikely to need repeating/redoing.

QUESTION 29: CONSENT

You see 45-year-old postman. He has been referred to Occupational Health because he has breached the absence threshold and it is the employer's policy to refer at this point. The referral states that he has multiple 1- or 2-day absences with 'viral illnesses'. He tells you in confidence that he has depression and is taking time off for counselling and on days when his motivation is low. He tells you that he does not want to lose his job and does not want a report to go to his employer. Despite your best efforts he will not give his consent for a report to be released.

The answer is: d) Without relevant information the employer can act on the information they have

Without information on any medical problem present (note – the diagnosis does not have to be revealed) then the employer does have a duty to provide reasonable adjustments if they reasonably presume that there is a need, but they can act on the information that they have (which is that he has taken multiple sick days for largely unknown reasons that appear to be unrelated), which may result in the termination of his contract. You can write to the employer to state that no report will be released as consent has been refused, but this is not as relevant given the wording of the question: 'he does not want to lose his job'. There are multiple reasons why people do not want to have details released – stigma being one of them.

QUESTION 30: REPORTS

You see a 56-year-old gentleman who works as a heavy goods vehicle (HGV) driver. He has been absent from work with bilateral knee and hip osteoarthritis for 6 months and has been referred to you for the first time, as management are concerned about the length of time he has had off work. He claims that he cannot climb in and out of the HGV. He is still driving a car and tells you that he can undertake the emergency stop procedure in both vehicles. He tells you that he is awaiting an arthroscopy of his right knee. On examination, the range of movement of his knee is moderately limited bilaterally with bilateral crepitus and he has a mildly antalgic gait.

The answer is: b) You should seek further information on his management from his treating doctor

It may be that his employer wishes to terminate his employment because he has breached the sickness absence threshold. Therefore it is important to get the facts as to whether he will be fit for the foreseeable future and if not, when his arthroscopy may be and his prognosis, as you do not have much clinical evidence to go on.

It is likely that he is fit to attend a capability meeting, but as this is not referred to in the statement, it is not the best answer.

QUESTION 31: BACK PAIN

You see a 20-year-old man who works as a carpenter in the boat-making industry. He is complaining of a twisting back injury after tripping 2 weeks ago. He has been off sick with back pain ever since. He has no red flags in his history, and on examination he has no neurology and a reasonable range of movement.

Regarding his return to work:

The answer is: b) He could return to work despite pain

Source: *Occupational Health Guidelines for the Management of Low Back Pain: evidence review and recommendations* (Waddell and Burton, 2000) Available via the Publications tab on the FOM website, www.fom.ac.uk

Active rehabilitation is important and as long as he is not on any painkillers with side-effects not conducive to work, he could return with small amounts of pain. A yellow flag, and poor prognostic indicator, would be a passive expectation of improvement or the idea that pain will be harmful to him. It is important to educate these patients, and the 'Back book' (www.nrmc.co.uk/wp-content/uploads/The-Back-Book.pdf) is a good educational tool. An accident analysis should be undertaken, but this will not aid his return to work, and a phased return may not be necessary.

QUESTION 32: DVLA

You see a 30-year-old student who had a witnessed loss of consciousness whilst sitting at his desk. The witness reportedly told him that he came around after a few seconds and he denies any prodromal symptoms and tells you that he was fully aware of himself and his surroundings when he regained consciousness. You look at the DVLA guidelines that state that he should not drive for one month and that he should inform the DVLA. He is adamant that it will not happen again and states that he will not drive if it happens again.

The answer is: d) Tell him that under no circumstances can he drive at present

The DVLA guidance is clear on this. The GMC guidelines state:

1) *The driver is legally responsible for informing the DVLA about such a condition or treatment. However, if a patient has such a condition, you should explain to the patient:*
   * *That the condition may affect their ability to drive (if the patient is incapable of understanding this advice, for example because of dementia, you should inform the DVLA immediately) and,*
   * *That they have a legal duty to inform the DVLA about the condition.*

2) *If a patient refuses to accept the diagnosis, or the effect of the condition on their ability to drive, you can suggest that they seek a second opinion, and help arrange for them to do so. You should advise the patient not to drive in the meantime.*

3) *If a patient continues to drive when they may not be fit to do so, you should make every reasonable effort to persuade them to stop. As long as the patient agrees, you may discuss your concerns with their relatives, friends or carers.*

4) *If you do not manage to persuade the patient to stop driving, or you discover that they are continuing to drive against your advice, you should contact the DVLA immediately and disclose any relevant medical information, in confidence, to the medical adviser.*

5) *Before contacting the DVLA, you should try to inform the patient of your decision to disclose personal information. You should also inform the patient in writing once you have done so.*

Whilst all of the above are relevant, and whilst some physicians may argue that it is appropriate to take the employee's keys, option (a) might be considered a bit extreme!

The bottom line is, he cannot continue to drive whilst he seeks a second opinion and breaking confidentiality is a last resort.

QUESTION 33: ACCESS TO MEDICAL RECORDS ACT

You discuss the outline of your report with an employee who wishes to see a copy of the report before it is sent to the employer.

The answer is: c) General Medical Council (GMC) guidance suggests that the patient should be allowed to see the report prior to the employer

The Access to Medical Records Act 1998 (AMRA) enables any individual to have the right to access their medical records for employment or insurance purposes. This applies to the treating physician. The Occupational Health Practitioner (OHP) is not the 'medical practitioner who is or has been responsible for the clinical care of the individual', therefore AMRA does not apply, but of most relevance is that it is FOM/BMA/GMC good practice to allow the prior viewing of the report. The other main difference is that the 21-day delay does not apply, and although it is not specified how long the patient has to read the report beforehand, most OH services allow between 2 and 5 days depending whether sent electronically or via post. If the individual does not reply within the time frame, then consent is assumed and the report sent to management. Confirmation of receipt by patient is not required. All patients should be allowed the opportunity to have prior viewing.

QUESTION 34: MENOPAUSE

You see a 54-year-old lady who has been referred after it was brought to management's attention that she was very irritable. She denied any problems with work or at home and any medical problems to management as part of a review because of this. Human Resources (HR) is asking you whether there is any medical problem to account for her behaviour and to advise if so on going forward to support her at work. She works as a receptionist in a busy hotel.

When you consult with her she tells you that she is going through the menopause and that she has been struggling with mood swings and difficulty sleeping for 2 months. She tells you that she did not want to discuss this with her line manager.

She consents for your report to be sent to her employer.

The answer is: c) You should advise HR that shift changes may be appropriate to help with sleeping difficulties

Source: *Guidance on Menopause and the Workplace* (FOM) Available at www.som.org.uk/sites/som.org.uk/files/Guidance-on-menopause-and-the-workplace.pdf

The FOM states that severe menopausal symptoms could fall under the Equality Act 2010. What are 'reasonable' adjustments is for the employer to decide, not for you; you can only make suggestions on medically necessary adjustments.

You could tell HR that she is menopausal, but as she does not want her manager to know then she may not want HR to know, and it would be better to provide as little clinical information as possible to make your point. In reality you would ask her if it was all right to disclose that she is menopausal.

QUESTION 35: DVLA

You see a driver of an 8-seater vehicle who had a stroke one month ago. He has no neurological deficit and is driving his car with no problem.

The employer has asked to know if he is fit to drive at work.

The answer is: b) As long as he has no neurological deficit he can drive an 8-seater vehicle

An 8-seater vehicle is a Group 1 vehicle and therefore he is able to drive this at work if he fits the criteria from the DVLA from one month after a stroke. He is not fit to drive a Group 2 vehicle, but this is not relevant to the question.

QUESTION 36: SHINGLES

You see a 60-year-old personal assistant to the chief executive of an advertising company who was diagnosed one week ago with shingles on her abdomen.

Work had insisted that she stays off work for one week, and also that she sees occupational health for advice before she can return to work.

The answer is: b) She can return to work with no restrictions

She can be at work if the condition can be covered. There is no risk to other employees as the lesions on the abdomen will be covered by routine clothing, thus no action for other staff needs to be taken.

QUESTION 37: CHICKENPOX

You are asked to see a 30-year-old bank Health Care Assistant who has come into contact with a patient two days before they developed disseminated shingles. She says that she has not had chickenpox. She is asymptomatic but worried.

The answer is: b) Her occupational health notes should show her immunisation status

Source: Varicella Zoster Virus: occupational aspects of management (RCP, 2010) Available at www.rcplondon.ac.uk/guidelines-policy/varicella-zoster-virus-occupational-aspects-management-2010

Varicella zoster virus vaccine is effective in providing adults with long-term protection from serious varicella zoster virus disease, and varicella zoster virus-susceptible healthcare workers should be offered vaccination using two doses of vaccine.

Healthcare workers diagnosed with localised herpes zoster on a part of the body that can be covered with a bandage and/or clothing should be allowed to work if they are clinically well. If they work with high-risk patients, an individual risk assessment should be carried out, to determine the appropriate action.

Susceptible healthcare workers who have a significant exposure to varicella zoster virus should either be excluded from contact with high-risk patients or inform their occupational health department if they feel unwell or develop a rash or fever during the incubation period. In general, elderly patients would not be considered high risk.

In the majority of situations a high level of vigilance for malaise, rash or fever (including taking temperature daily) throughout the incubation period will be adequate.

QUESTION 38: UPPER LIMB DISORDERS

Mr Dale is a 24-year-old picker in a toy warehouse. For the last 3 months he tells you that he has had pain in his right forearm and elbow. He is left-handed. In his spare time he plays darts, but has not been able to do so because of the pain. He is otherwise fit and well. On abduction of the elbow against resistance he complains of pain. You know that other packers have similar symptoms and suspect that the organisation needs to undertake a risk assessment.

The answer is: d) Assessing neck pain is appropriate

The term 'upper limb disorders' includes neck pain.

A questionnaire can be a quick and easy way of assessing general risk and prioritising your assessment.

Once a risk assessment has been undertaken, it is useful to involve those 'on the ground' in suggesting control measures – this helps to create a safety culture. Look at whether practically the controls will be appropriate; this could involve further training.

There is no specific legislation relating to upper limb disorders, but this is not the most appropriate answer in relation to risk assessments.

QUESTION 39: DIABETES

You are asked to see a district nurse to advise on any adjustments needed to her work as a result of her ongoing pregnancy. She is 30/40. She has gestational diabetes and has been started on insulin one month ago, with no complications so far. She is otherwise well and her blood sugars have been stable. Driving is integral to her role.

Regarding advice you should give her and her employer:

The answer is: d) Her employer must undertake a risk assessment now that she is pregnant

She can drive as long as she is not at risk from 'disabling hypoglycaemia', which the question suggests. She does not need to inform the DVLA if she is going to be on insulin transiently (less than 3 months), which is likely to be the case. The employer should undertake a new risk assessment as her medical status has changed.

QUESTION 40: DIABETES

You are asked to see a poorly controlled type 2 diabetic who is a trainee paramedic, for an opinion on fitness for her role. She is not on insulin, but tells you that her consultant has advised her that she may need to be 'in the future'.

The answer is: b) She will be subject to yearly DVLA checks to confirm her fitness to drive an ambulance

Insulin-treated diabetics can drive ambulances, under certain circumstances.

Shift working can upset glucose control due to the timing of insulin doses if control has not been established.

QUESTION 41: NEEDLE-STICK INJURIES

You consult with a frantic junior doctor who has just obtained a needle-stick injury from a patient in A and E. The donor has just died.

The next line of management by occupational health would be to:

The answer is: b) Start post-exposure prophylaxis

Consent is needed from a relative to take blood from a deceased donor.

A needle-stick injury is not RIDDOR reportable.

No restrictions on practice are needed.

QUESTION 42: ALCOHOL

You are in clinic when a junior doctor asks for some urgent advice. She thinks that her consultant is drunk because he is acting oddly and she smelt alcohol on his breath.

She does not know what to do.

The answer is: a) The consultant is not fit for work, with immediate effect

He is not fit to work at the moment and transport should be arranged to get him home. The concern at this point is that patient safety is potentially at risk. Immediate testing is frequently normally advised by a designated individual, not Occupational Health, as set out in the employer's policy, and a review by Occupational Health at a later date would be appropriate.

QUESTION 43: UPPER LIMB DISORDERS

You see a 35-year-old administrator who complains of pain in her right elbow which is worse on most movements and appears to be aggravated by long periods of time typing on the computer. She is able to undertake activities outside of work, but finds that after an hour of being at work her symptoms get worse. She tells you that she has tried wrist splints, non-steroidal anti-inflammatory drugs (NSAIDs) and physiotherapy, and is keen to have any other suggestions.

The answer is: a) There is no specific legislation directly related to upper limb disorders

She does not display any yellow or red flags, which are an indicator of a worse outcome, and is unlikely to be exposed to significant vibration effects as an administrator, so these statements are not as relevant, despite being correct. The employer has a duty to provide reasonable adjustments.

QUESTION 44: HOME WORKING

You see a 45-year-old data manager who is recovering from chemotherapy. As part of his return to work plan he has requested to work at home for 2 days a week. The employer has approved this request.

The answer is: b) Employers have a duty to apply the same health and safety standards to home workers as those in the workplace

The most relevant principle is that, when looking at the risks to the employee and others, the same standards that apply at work apply at home.

QUESTION 45: MENTAL HEALTH

You see a carpenter in a large construction site who tells you that he is feeling low. He tells you that 2 months ago he tried to commit suicide by hanging himself, but was found by his girlfriend. He tells you that he has been at work since this event (work are not aware of it) and that he is being followed up by the crisis team once a week. He tells you that as far as he is aware, there are no concerns from management about the quality of his work. His role involves working at height, working alone, and working with moving part machinery.

Regarding the next management step to take:

The answer is: b) He should not undertake lone working

He is 2 months after the event and under intermittent review from the crisis team, suggesting that his risk is lower than it was 2 months ago. He has been working throughout his ill health with no apparent issues and therefore putting him on sickness absence could be considered extreme. Lowering the risk at work would involve removing him from lone working, and in this time you could write to his mental health team.

QUESTION 46: HUMAN IMMUNODEFICIENCY VIRUS (HIV)

You undertake a pre-employment consultation with Mr Bleasdale, a 32-year-old man applying for a role at Maydie Hospital as a porter. He discloses that he is HIV positive, with a CD4 count over 400, and no other medical problems. At present he is not on antiviral therapy due to problems with unacceptable side-effects, but is due to see his consultant for a review of medications in 2 months. He has a past history of carpal tunnel syndrome, for which he wears splints at night, and has a history of epilepsy. He is on 500 mg of Keppra, and his last fit was 2 months ago, when he had three fits in one week.

Regarding what you should inform Human Resources of:

The answer is: e) He should not undertake lone working

With a history of uncontrolled epilepsy he should not undertake lone working, but his disclosure of his HIV status is not a barrier to working in a hospital, nor is there any current need for you to talk with him about disclosing to his prospective employer, because his CD4 count is good and he has no side-effects from medication.

QUESTION 47: CARDIOLOGY

An employee has cardiac trouble and has a pacemaker fitted, then returns unannounced, appearing on site back at work one day where electromagnetic fields are present. The manager both phones and emails you in a panic, asking if the individual is fit for work and whether or not they can stay on site; are they fit for work and can they stay on site?

The answer is: c) Place him on medical suspension until you can obtain the answer

An OHP would not be expected to know the answer off the top of their head, but they would be expected to know how and where to get information in order to come to the correct decision. In the meantime, the individual should be medically suspended pending a decision being made, or provided with tasks in an area that is guaranteed to have no electromagnetic field (EMF) exposures whatsoever.

Each pacemaker is different and each patient is informed of both the manufacturer and serial number. From these, the manufacturer needs to be contacted regarding their guidance on absolute EMF exposure and, if permitted, level of EMF exposure without detriment to either patient and/or pacemaker. It is likely that the manufacturer will respond with yes/no to EMF and, if so, the individual cannot be exposed to high levels of EMF – with "high" not further elaborated upon.

The Consultant Cardiologist needs to be written to (no AMRA consent is needed) to ask them what their definition of "high" EMF exposure would be, in association with pacemaker brand and serial number.

The onsite Health and Safety team need to provide you with (or go and measure it for the first time!) the exact kind of EMF and quantity of EMF at every location, including toilets/canteen/car park/reception/meeting rooms/training rooms, as well as actual job locations, on site at which the individual might in any way conceivably be located at any given time.

QUESTION 48: DIABETES

A type 2 diabetic taxi driver has been referred to you for advice regarding fitness to drive and depression, and when you ask him about his medication he mentions that he was started on insulin 2 months ago for his diabetes.

Regarding his driving:

The answer is: d) His ability to drive in the future will be subject to a yearly assessment by a consultant in diabetic medicine

The DVLA 'Fitness to drive' guidance recommends that taxi drivers should meet the same medical standards that Group 2 bus and lorry drivers must meet under the DVLA's requirements. Therefore he is subject to a yearly review by a consultant diabetologist/endocrinologist as part of his licensing procedure, as set out in the guidelines for Group 2 drivers. Therefore he does need to inform the DVLA regardless for many reasons, but the most important is not his insurance! Also, it is important to note that he needs to stop driving immediately until he is approved to drive any class of vehicle by the DVLA.

Under the Equality Act 2010 direct discrimination would occur if insurance companies had higher tariffs on the basis of their diagnosis alone.

QUESTION 49: ILL HEALTH RETIREMENT

You see a 45-year-old teaching assistant who has applied for ill heath retirement. She tells you that she has arthritis of her left hip and is finding mobilising around a classroom and between classrooms painful. She describes her walking as slow, and feels that she does not want to disadvantage the children she helps by leaving the classroom early to get to her next class, but if she does not do this then she feels unable to walk fast enough to get to her next lesson on time. She comes with a supporting letter from her head teacher, which states that he is unable to accommodate any reduction in hours or change her working schedule so that her classes are closer together, nor can he provide a wheelchair; he feels that she needs ill health retirement as she clearly cannot work in her condition, and as a valued member of staff would have to be made redundant. On examination she walks with a three wheeler aid, is very slow to mobilise, has difficulty getting in and out of a chair, and is morbidly obese.

The answer is: c) You should suggest that weight reduction could enable her to work

Generally an application for ill health retirement requires that the employee be unable to continue with their job for medical reasons, having exhausted all treatment options or no treatment option being able to help her work.

In this case she could lose weight, which would potentially help with all these problems to an extent that she could work.

QUESTION 50: BACK PAIN

You see a 34-year-old carpenter who suffers from recurrent low back pain. He has no red flag symptoms or signs. His examination is limited by pain. He does not take any analgesia as he 'does not like to take medication'. He tells you that this episode was exacerbated by a work episode where he had to lift a heavy door by himself. You have noticed an increasing incidence of back pain in workers in his department.

The answer is: a) An ergonomics assessment takes into account organisational factors

This employee (and perhaps the others in his department) needs an ergonomics assessment of their environment. It may be that organisational factors may play a part – for example an unrealistic expectation of tasks to be completed, or poor attitude to safety.

The Assessment of Repetitive Tasks (ART) is for assessing upper limb disorders.

It may be that manual handling refresher training is needed, but this needs to be assessed in the ergonomic risk assessment.

QUESTION 51: SAFEGUARDING

You see a sales assistant who has been referred with depression. She is a single mum and looks unkempt. You think that she has severe depression. On her way out, you notice that she has left her 2-year-old daughter on her own in the waiting room. You observe that the girl looks malnourished and dirty and you feel there is the potential that she has been neglected.

The answer is: b) A referral to social services for safeguarding issues can be made without consent

Answer E is also correct.

In this case you should speak to a safeguarding expert. In the absence of this advice you should refer to social services.

An OHP may need to consider safeguarding issues when an employee may be suffering from a condition that could potentially put a child at risk.

www.fom.ac.uk/wp-content/uploads/FOM-RCPCH-Safeguarding-Children-Guidelines-for-OHPs.pdf

QUESTION 52: PRE-EMPLOYMENT SCREENING

Ms Smith has applied for job as an administrator on an obstetric ward. She has refused a complete screening test to check her varicella zoster virus status and declares that she has not had chickenpox.

The answer is: a) Check that she has been properly informed as to why the test is needed

Answers C and E are also correct.

She should be given the opportunity to have all the information before refusing a test, as the employer cannot be obliged to risk employing her without this data.

QUESTION 53: BIOLOGICAL MONITORING

Regarding biological monitoring:

The answer is: a) Consent is always needed to take samples for monitoring

Source: www.hse.gov.uk/pubns/books/hsg167.htm

- **Health guidance value (HGV).** HGVs are set at a level at which there is no indication from the scientific evidence available that the substance being monitored is likely to be injurious to health. Values not greatly in excess of an HGV are unlikely to produce serious short- or long-term effects on health. However, regularly exceeding the HGV does indicate that control of exposure may not be adequate. Under these circumstances employers will need to look at current work practices to see how they can be improved to reduce exposure.
- **Benchmark guidance value (BGV).** BGVs are not health-based. They are practicable, achievable levels set at the 90th percentile of available biological monitoring results collected from a representative sample of workplaces with good occupational hygiene practices. If a result is greater than a BGV it does not necessarily mean that ill health will occur, but it does indicate that control of exposure may not be adequate. Under these circumstances employers will need to look at current work practices to see how they can be improved to reduce exposure.

QUESTION 54: HAND ARM VIBRATION SYNDROME (HAVS)

A 30-year-old shipbuilder presents with intermittent tingling and blanching in his left hand. He works with many vibrating tools. He has a family history of systemic lupus erythematosus (his mum). He has a marked left-sided tremor (in his left hand only). He has reduced power globally in his left forearm. Fine motor movements were normal. Purdue test was normal and monofilament tests were normal also. Phalen's and Tinel's are unremarkable.

Regarding the next option in managing this employee:

The answer is: a) Advise a GP review

This picture is suspicious of a neurological problem that is not vibration-related. He may have HAVS as a separate diagnosis.
A GP review is warranted to rule out other neurological problems.

The diagnosis of HAVS is secondary to this, but would involve a risk assessment and proof of hand blanching.

QUESTION 55: MISCELLANEOUS

You see a professor of physics who has been referred after complaining of 'exhaustion'. She tells you that she has just finished a project that she has found challenging and has also had to manage two colleagues who have not been getting on.

She denies that she is 'stressed'. She tells you that she has had reduced sleep but no other symptoms.

Her employer wants advice regarding the best way of avoiding a relapse of her symptoms.

The answer is: c) Reducing job demands could help

She has told you that she does not feel stressed and so is unlikely to be willing to fill in a stress risk assessment form. Whilst a controversial topic, work-related stress is common and the HSE acknowledges five controllable variables that will help reduce it. She is telling you that she has had a difficult personnel issue to manage, as well as feeling challenged at work, and therefore C is the best answer.

QUESTION 56: TOURETTE'S SYNDROME

You see a 35-year-old lecturer with Tourette's syndrome. He is facing a disciplinary for offensive behaviour, as there have been several complaints about comments he has made (possibly as part of his syndrome); as part of a management plan has been referred to occupational health.

Regarding the advice you should give:

The answer is: b) Controlling his outbursts is a management issue

Outbursts cannot be controlled, and have PR and management implications; therefore management need to decide what to do about the nature of the outbursts and any sequelae that occur as a result of them. This can be a capability issue if problems continue to occur.

QUESTION 57: UPPER LIMB DISORDERS

You see an administrator who complains of pain and numbness in the thumb and first finger of her right hand. She thinks that her symptoms only occur at work whilst she is typing. A workstation assessment has been undertaken before she sees you, but she tells you that a split keyboard and penguin mouse have not helped. She feels that her symptoms are getting worse. Tinel's and Phalen's tests are negative. She is becoming less productive and management are keen to know what help may be available for her.

The answer is: b) Referral to occupational therapist

Basic principles apply here: conservative before medical or surgical. An OT can advise on the type of splint (e.g. resting or working) that may be appropriate. NSAIDs are not used in the course of management of carpal tunnel syndrome. The other options are less relevant in a case of mild carpal tunnel syndrome.

NICE CKS and guidelines for healthcare commissioning from BSSH, BOA and RCS Eng suggest that patients with mild CTS should improve within 6 weeks of non-surgical management (with splint and corticosteroid injection).

QUESTION 58: BLUE LIGHT DRIVING

You have seen a stable insulin-dependent diabetic policewoman with an HbA1c of 65. She has had a car accident where the matter of her fitness to drive police vehicles is being questioned.

The answer is: d) An individual decision can be made at the discretion of the Force Medical Adviser

Source: www.fom.ac.uk/wp-content/uploads/FOM-Guide-re-blue-light-driving.pdf

The DVLA suggests that those with insulin-treated diabetes should not drive emergency vehicles, and blue light driving is referred to by the DVLA in its document "At a Glance" which then goes on to state that the advice on interpreting these recommendations should be undertaken in the knowledge of specific circumstance (an individual risk assessment approach) including patient factors, the frequency of the driving and type of vehicle.

The FOM suggests that for any vehicles that drive outside of the normal traffic laws, Group 2 standards are used. For those that follow the normal traffic rules (such as unmarked cars) Group 1 standards can be used.

The FOM suggests that for those individuals who do not meet the Group 2 guidance (driving under blue lights), an OHP familiar with the job role can undertake a risk assessment approach, known as the "Group 2 minus" approach. This needs to take into account factors such as motivation, other co-morbidities and the duration of the condition.

QUESTION 59: EPILEPSY

Regarding the maximum level of annual risk of sustaining a seizure accepted for holding a Group 2 driving licence:

The answer is: a) 2%

20% is the maximum level of annual risk of sustaining a seizure accepted for holding a Group 1 licence.

QUESTION 60: NOISE

Health and Safety perform a risk assessment of a factory and identify that the noise levels are too high.

Regarding the most appropriate form of control:

The answer is: a) Anti-vibration mounting under machinery

Engineering controls are more effective in the hierarchy of control.

PPE is always a last resort.

Health surveillance is not a form of control.

References and resources

British Occupational Health Research Foundation: www.bohrf.org.uk [last accessed 11 April 2017]

Connelly, P. *Presbycusis – A Look into the Aging Inner Ear*. International Hearing Society. Available at: www.ihsinfo.org/IhsV2/hearing_professional/2003/060_November-December/080_Presbycusis_A_Look_into_the_Aging_Inner_Ear.cfm [last accessed 11 April 2017]

Driver and Vehicle Licensing Agency: www.gov.uk/government/organisations/driver-and-vehicle-licensing-agency [last accessed 11 April 2017]

General Medical Council: www.gmc-uk.org [last accessed 11 April 2017]

Health and Safety Executive: www.hse.gov.uk [last accessed 11 April 2017]

Healthy Working Lives: www.healthyworkinglives.com [last accessed 11 April 2017]

Smedley, J., Dick, F. and Sadhra, S. (2013) *Oxford Handbook of Occupational Health*, 2nd edition. Oxford: Oxford University Press.